Collaborative Drug Therapy Management Handbook

Sarah A. Tracy, Pharm.D., BCPS

Clinical Pharmacist and Clinical Projects Coordinator
Harborview Medical Center
Seattle, Washington
Clinical Assistant Professor
University of Washington School of Pharmacy

Cynthia A. Clegg, B.S. Pharm., M.H.A.

Supervisor, Ambulatory Pharmacy Services
Harborview Medical Center
Seattle, Washington
Clinical Associate Professor
University of Washington School of Pharmacy

American Society of Health-System Pharmacists®
Bethesda, Maryland

Any correspondence regarding this publication should be sent to the publisher, American Society of Health-System Pharmacists, 7272 Wisconsin Avenue, Bethesda, MD 20814, attention: Special Publishing.

The information presented herein reflects the opinions of the contributors and advisors. It should not be interpreted as an official policy of ASHP or as an endorsement of any product.

Because of ongoing research and improvements in technology, the information and its applications contained in this text are constantly evolving and are subject to the professional judgment and interpretation of the practitioner due to the uniqueness of a clinical situation. The editors, contributors, and ASHP have made reasonable efforts to ensure the accuracy and appropriateness of the information presented in this document. However, any user of this information is advised that the editors, contributors, advisors, and ASHP are not responsible for the continued currency of the information, for any errors or omissions, and/or for any consequences arising from the use of the information in the document in any and all practice settings. Any reader of this document is cautioned that ASHP makes no representation, guarantee, or warranty, express or implied, as to the accuracy and appropriateness of the information contained in this document and specifically disclaims any liability to any party for the accuracy and/or completeness of the material or for any damages arising out of the use or non-use of any of the information contained in this document.

Director, Special Publishing: Jack Bruggeman
Acquisitions Editor: Hal Pollard
Senior Editorial Project Manager: Dana Battaglia
Production Editor: Johnna Hershey
Cover/Page Design and Composition: David Wade

Library of Congress Cataloging-in-Publication Data

Collaborative drug therapy management handbook / [edited by] Sarah A. Tracy, Cynthia A. Clegg.
    p. ; cm.
 ISBN 978-1-58528-160-2
 1. Pharmacy--Practice--Handbooks, manuals, etc. 2.
Drugs--Prescribing--Handbooks, manuals, etc. I. Tracy, Sarah A. II. Clegg,
Cynthia A. III. American Society of Health-System Pharmacists.
 [DNLM: 1. Drug Therapy--Handbooks. 2. Patient Care Team--Handbooks. WB
39 C697 2007]
 RS100.3.C65 2007
 615'.1--dc22
                        2007025779

ISBN: 978-1-58528-160-2

Dedication

To Cindi Brennan

"Leadership is the capacity to translate vision into reality."
-Warren G. Bennis

Foreword

The passage of the Medicare Prescription Drug Improvement and Modernization Act in 2003 (Public Law 108-173) has created significant opportunities for pharmacists. This was a landmark piece of legislation that called for the establishment of medication therapy management programs designed to reduce the risk of adverse events and optimize therapeutic outcomes through improved medication use. The law allows for the convergence of the medication therapy needs of patients and the unique clinical skills of pharmacists. However, there has been reluctance on the part of some pharmacists to participate in these programs due to workload pressures, reimbursement issues, and the lack of skills necessary to implement and sustain these programs.

As the current demand for health care professionals exceeds the existing supply and is in turn coupled with escalating health care costs, where can pharmacists provide the greatest value? How will our profession be able to balance safety and affordability and at the same time provide care to the nearly 47 million uninsured Americans? How can we best participate in health promotion and improve quality of life for our patients? While pharmacists are responsible for the overall pharmacy enterprise, it is imperative that we fully engage in both clinical and non-clinical activities that promote safe and cost-effective use of medications. This will include delegating the technical aspects of pharmacy operations to technicians who, when properly trained, will set a new standard in our profession. We believe that engaging pharmacists in providing evidence-based collaborative patient care will enhance patient safety, bring about desired outcomes, and propel our profession to become *the* medication-use experts. This practice model empowers pharmacists to integrate evidence-based medicine and patient-centered care, which reduces the gap between best science and actual prescribing practices.

The first edition of the *Collaborative Drug Therapy Management Handbook* provides a framework for designing, developing, implementing, and sustaining an evidence-based approach to achieving the desired outcomes in the ambulatory arena. It is a practical guide for leading pharmacists, clinical coordinators, and pharmacy administrators in the successful creation of new clinical programs. The book is written by one of the finest groups of dedicated pharmacist professionals who excel each day in providing optimal patient care while simultaneously participating in teaching and research. Many of these pharmacists practice in primary care clinics, where they work side by side with other health care providers to manage multiple disease states in the provision of patient-centered care. The chapters in this book capture the daily work and expertise of these clinicians. The cornerstones of primary care are represented, as are several specialty areas in which we manage medication therapy. Select case studies provide practical application of the concepts presented. In addition, this handbook provides information on credentialing and outcomes collection and reporting, both which serve to strongly support collaborative drug therapy management.

Patient-centered clinical care has evolved at Harborview Medical Center over the past 20 years. Harborview is managed by the University of Washington; it is Seattle's county hospital and the Pacific Northwest region's only Level I trauma center. It faces similar issues to other county hospitals around the country with the teaching and research mission common to all academic institutions. The interdisciplinary collaborative services presented in this handbook are a result of the vision and tenacity of Cindi Brennan, Assistant Director of Ambulatory Pharmacy Services at Harborview Medical Center, with strong support from Drew Edwards, Director of Pharmacy Operations, and Cyndy Clegg, Ambulatory Pharmacy Services Supervisor. Over the years, tremendous energy has been spent working with hospital administration, as well as medical, nursing, and pharmacy staff in advancing evidence-based pharmacy services. Physician opinion leaders were enlisted to help promote the value of pharmacists in positively affecting patient outcomes and thereby help physicians increase their productivity through pharmacist-managed drug therapy. In addition, pharmacists were engaged in the development of protocols, house-staff education, and research. These services, along with the Pharmacy Department's ability to significantly contain medication costs, resulted in the establishment of the role of the pharmacist as a medication therapy manager.

Shabir M. Somani, M.S., M.B.A., R.Ph., FASHP
Director of Pharmacy Services, University of Washington Medical Center
Harborview Medical Center, Seattle Cancer Care Alliance
Professor, University of Washington School of Pharmacy

Preface

The practice of collaborative drug therapy management (CDTM) began at the Harborview Medical Center (HMC) Pharmacy Department many years ago. It started with one pharmacist, a medication cart, and a typewriter (see *Introduction* chapter). Today, the HMC pharmacy has pharmacists in all primary care and most specialty clinics.

This handbook represents years of experience and practice in CDTM. It is intended for any pharmacist or administrator seeking to initiate, improve, or expand CDTM services in his or her organization. It is designed as a starting point for establishing collaborative practice, and is not in any way meant to serve as a complete therapeutic reference.

Three major sections are included in this reference book: the introduction, example guidelines, and quality assurance mechanisms.

The introduction provides a brief background and presents the core elements necessary for establishing a CDTM program.

The example guidelines were created by our team of outstanding clinical pharmacy specialists and are used in our daily practice at Harborview Medical Center. They may be utilized in their current format or adjusted as needed for your particular institution. We are fortunate to have a very liberal practice environment, and as a result the guidelines are quite general and provide flexibility for considerable clinician judgment. Other practice sites may require more specific stepwise protocols. The guidelines are subdivided into *Indications, Management, Goals of Therapy, Clinical Pharmacy Goals, Outcome Measures, Patient Information Resources* (and in some chapters, *Provider Resources*), and a *Case Study*. The section entitled *Indications* provides information on identifying eligible patients; *Management* presents guidelines for pharmacologic and non-pharmacologic treatment of the specified disease state; *Goals of Therapy* lists treatment goals; *Clinical Pharmacy Goals* identifies objectives the clinical pharmacist should address in the treatment process; *Outcome Measures* offers examples of outcomes divided among process measures, surrogate markers, and health outcomes measures corresponding to the discussion in the chapter discussing outcomes; *Patient Information Resources* lists information sources suitable for patient reference; and the case studies contained in many chapters serve to illustrate the application of the CDTM guidelines in clinical practice. The thought process behind the decisions is indicated in the plan in italics.

The chapters on quality assurance include information on pharmacist privileging and measuring outcomes. The privileging process is necessary for verifying the credentials of clinical pharmacists and is an important step in ensuring that patients receive quality care. The outcomes chapter provides information on various outcome measures and the utility of each. The collection of outcomes is essential for evaluating the success of a CDTM program, in addition to addressing areas for improvement.

As pharmacy practice continues to evolve with a greater focus on cognitive services and medication therapy management (MTM), CDTM is becoming increasingly important and widespread. We hope this handbook is a useful resource for any pharmacist interested or involved in CDTM.

Sarah A. Tracy
Cynthia A. Clegg
May 2007

Acknowledgments

The publication of this handbook has been a challenging and rewarding journey. We are indebted first and foremost to Cindi Brennan for her vision of clinical pharmacy practice in the days long before anyone had thought to pen the phrase "collaborative drug therapy management." Her leadership and passion for the profession has created clinical practice at Harborview Medical Center that is recognized nationally as a model of exemplary patient care. We owe a great deal of our success to Dan Lessler, our physician champion. When Dan first met Cindi in 1993, he said, "Glad to meet you. Now, where are my Pharm.D.s?" His ongoing support and influence with the medical staff has helped to create an environment that supports the highest level of collaborative practice.

An incredible amount of gratitude is owed to the clinical pharmacist specialists who labored beyond their daily clinical practices to create clear and succinct synopses of their practice specialties. These experts were committed to producing a quality product that will enhance and advance the profession of pharmacy.

Many thanks to Carol Crawford, Katie Lai, Chelsea Newport, Cathy Null, David Roesel, and Ann Wittkowsky for their participation in the peer review process and for providing expertise.

We are grateful for the guidance of the Harborview Pharmacy Administration team: Shabir Somani, Drew Edwards, Cindi Brennan, Beverly Sheridan, and Cindy Wilson. We wish to thank Cindy Hecker, our Associate Administrator, and Johnese Spisso, Clinical Operations Officer, UW Medicine and Vice President of Medical Affairs, University of Washington, for their strong support of the department of pharmacy.

The ambulatory pharmacy staff at Harborview is an extraordinary group. Their commitment to the mission of the organization is evidenced every day through their ongoing provision of clinical and distributive services.

ASHP provided tremendous encouragement and assistance in the preparation of this handbook. We first discussed the project with Hal Pollard in 2005. He shared our vision, and his enthusiasm was contagious. Throughout the drafting and editing process, Dana Battaglia provided almost daily support to us and was an invaluable resource. We greatly appreciate Hal, Dana, Johnna Hershey, and others at ASHP who were instrumental in making this handbook a reality.

Professionally, I (CAC) am very fortunate to have spent the majority of my career working with Cindi Brennan. She has been an extraordinary mentor and friend. Personally, I am deeply grateful for the support of my family. My mother, Dorothy, has been the consummate role model and has always encouraged me to strive to make a difference in the world. And my sons, Matthew and Ethan, remind me every day of the rich blessings in my life.

I (SAT) am indebted to Cindi Brennan, Cyndy Clegg, Tim Ives, and Terry Seaton who have all been instrumental in my professional development. I am extremely thankful for the support of my family. My husband, Chris, is my rock and encourages all of my endeavors. My parents, Phil and Vicki, and our nanny, Andy, provided the much needed childcare so my work on this handbook could be completed. My children, Anna and Owen, make each day an adventure and help me savor every moment and enjoy the little things in life.

Sarah A. Tracy
Cynthia A. Clegg
Editors

Table of Contents

Contributors

Harborview Medical Center Team
Seattle, Washington

Manzi Berlin, Pharm.D.
Clinical Pharmacist
Clinical Instructor
University of Washington School of Pharmacy

Cynthia A. Clegg, B.S. Pharm., M.H.A.
Supervisor, Ambulatory Pharmacy Services
Clinical Associate Professor
University of Washington School of Pharmacy

Karen Crabb, B.S. Pharm.
Clinical Pharmacist
Clinical Instructor
University of Washington School of Pharmacy

Vicki DeCaro, Pharm.D.
Clinical Pharmacist
Clinical Instructor
University of Washington School of Pharmacy

Tiffany Erickson, Pharm.D., BCPS
Clinical Pharmacist
Clinical Instructor
University of Washington School of Pharmacy

Alvin Goo, Pharm.D.
Clinical Pharmacist
Clinical Assistant Professor
University of Washington School of Pharmacy

Laura J. Hanson, Pharm.D., BCPS, CDE
Clinical Pharmacist
Clinical Assistant Professor
University of Washington School of Pharmacy

Beth Hykes, Pharm.D.
Clinical Pharmacist
Clinical Assistant Professor
University of Washington School of Pharmacy

Carol Johnson, B.S. Pharm.
Clinical Pharmacist
Clinical Assistant Professor
University of Washington School of Pharmacy

Jennifer Kapur, Pharm.D.
Clinical Pharmacist
Clinical Assistant Professor
University of Washington School of Pharmacy

Mary Sturgeleski Kelly, Pharm.D.
Clinical Pharmacist
Clinical Assistant Professor
University of Washington School of Pharmacy

Ji Eun Lee, Pharm.D., BCPS
Clinical Pharmacist
Clinical Instructor
University of Washington School of Pharmacy

Theresa O'Young, Pharm.D.
Clinical Pharmacist
Clinical Assistant Professor
University of Washington School of Pharmacy

Elaine Pappas, Pharm.D., BCPS
Clinical Pharmacist
Clinical Assistant Professor
University of Washington School of Pharmacy

Steve Riddle, B.S. Pharm., BCPS
Lead Pharmacist
Medication Utilization and Quality Improvement
Clinical Assistant Professor
University of Washington School of Pharmacy

Myrna Romack, B.S. Pharm.
Clinical Pharmacist
Clinical Assistant Professor
University of Washington School of Pharmacy

Heidi Sawyer, Pharm.D., BCPS
Clinical Pharmacist

Stephen Strockbine, B.S. Pharm.
Clinical Pharmacist
Clinical Assistant Professor
University of Washington School of Pharmacy

Greta Sweney, B.S. Pharm., BCPS
Clinical Pharmacist
Clinical Assistant Professor
University of Washington School of Pharmacy

Sarah A. Tracy, Pharm.D., BCPS
Clinical Pharmacist and Clinical Projects Coordinator
Clinical Assistant Professor
University of Washington School of Pharmacy

Marianne Weber, Pharm.D., BCPS
Clinical Pharmacist
Clinical Instructor
University of Washington School of Pharmacy

Carrie L. Yuan, Pharm.D., BCPS
Clinical Pharmacist
Clinical Instructor
University of Washington School of Pharmacy

Introduction to Collaborative Drug Therapy Management

Sarah A. Tracy **INTRODUCTION**

The practice of pharmacy has evolved from a profession whose sole purpose was to distribute pharmaceutical products to one that relies upon the pharmacist's unique expertise to help patients best utilize their medication. This practice model, known as collaborative drug therapy management (CDTM), is a team approach to health care delivery that focuses the pharmacist's attention on the patient's health-related needs. When participating in CDTM, pharmacists share the responsibility for patient outcomes. With this model, pharmacists solve patient- and medication-related problems and make decisions regarding drug prescribing, monitoring, and drug regimen adjustments, in addition to providing basic dispensing functions and drug information services.[1]

Pharmacist involvement in drug therapy management leads to improved medication safety, enhanced patient care, and lower medical costs. CDTM agreements make the provision of this care more accessible and effective because the pharmacist is able to directly impact patient care and clinical outcomes.

Definitions

ASHP defines CDTM as follows:

Collaborative drug therapy management is a multidisciplinary process for selecting appropriate drug therapies, educating patients, monitoring patients, and continually assessing outcomes of therapy. Collaborative drug therapy management is initiated after a patient receives a confirmed diagnosis by an authorized prescriber. The pharmacist, with the patient's other health care providers, then collaborates to effectively manage the patient's drug therapy. Collaborative drug therapy management may include but is not limited to: initiating, modifying, and monitoring a patient's drug therapy; ordering and performing laboratory and related tests; assessing patient response to

1

therapy; counseling and educating a patient on medications; and administering medications.[2]

The American College of Clinical Pharmacy (ACCP) defines CDTM by pharmacists as:

A collaborative practice agreement between one or more physicians and pharmacists wherein qualified pharmacists working within the context of a defined protocol are permitted to assume professional responsibility for performing patient assessments; ordering drug therapy-related laboratory tests; administering drugs; and selecting, initiating, monitoring, continuing, and adjusting drug regimens.[3]

History of Collaborative Drug Therapy Management Legislation

Federal legislation defers authority for determining pharmacist scope of practice to individual states. Authority for CDTM is generally incorporated in state pharmacy practice acts within the definition section describing pharmacists' scope of practice. There is no standard format for state pharmacy practice acts. Therefore, collaborative agreements vary significantly based on the type of agreement, required level of review or approval, medications, practice environment, and pharmacist education and training requirements (**Table 1**).

In the 1960s and 1970s, pharmacists began to assume roles as direct patient care providers in rural areas within the Indian Health Service. It was in this setting that the activity of pharmacist prescribing was first documented. In 1972, individual states began exploring the issue of pharmacist prescribing. California and Washington were the first states to implement CDTM programs. The 1997 ACCP position statement provides details of these early CDTM experiences.[1] The number of states with legislation or regulations authorizing pharmacists to engage in CDTM has increased substantially, especially over the past decade. As of early 2007, 43 states allowed various types of CDTM within their pharmacist scope of practice (**Figure 1**).

Prescriptive authority is not required in order to perform many of the duties involved in selecting, initiating, monitoring, continuing, modifying, and administering drug therapy. Nor is the ability to initiate drug therapy a prerequisite condition for pharmacists to establish a therapeutic relationship with a patient, solve drug-related problems, assume responsibility for therapeutic outcomes, or improve a patient's quality of life. However, when legally available, initiating drug regimen changes through CDTM agreements makes provision of care easier, more efficient, and convenient.[1]

Obstacles and Requirements for Establishing CDTM

Many pharmacists, even those in states that have legislative approval, do not currently engage in CDTM because of various obstacles. These obstacles include:

List of States by Statutory and Regulatory Authority
(Updated August 2006)

STATE	CDTM	STATUTE	REGULATION	PRACTICE SETTING	2005-2006 ACTIVITY
Alabama			PENDING		
Alaska	X		X	All	
Arizona	X	X	X	HC Institutions: Hospitals; Staff Models of a Health Care Organization; Nursing Care Institution; Community Health Center	
Arkansas	X	X	X	All	
California	X	X		All	
Colorado	X		X	All	3 CCR 719-1 6.00.00
Connecticut	X	X		Hospital Inpatients, Long Term Care Facilities	
Delaware		PENDING			
District of Columbia					
Florida	X	X		All (By Formulary)	
Georgia	X	X		All	
Hawaii	X	X		Licensed Acute Care Hospitals and ambulatory settings.	
Idaho	X		X	All	
Illinois[1]	X			All	
Indiana	X	X		Acute Care Settings; Private Mental Health Institutions	
Iowa[2]	X			Retail and health-system pharmacies that meet eligibility requirements for the Medicaid Demonstration Project (see footnote).	
Kansas[3]	X			All	
Kentucky	X	X	X	All	
Louisiana	X	X	X	All	
Maine					
Maryland	X	X		Institutional Facility (not included a nursing facility or an unrelated Urgent Care Clinic)	
Massachusetts		PENDING			
Michigan[4]	X			All	
Minnesota	X	X		All	
Mississippi	X	X	X	Institutional Settings; Outpatient Settings (must be signed protocol for each patient)	
Missouri					
Montana	X	X		All	
Nebraska	X	X		All	
Nevada	X	X		Licensed Medical Facilities: Hospitals; Hospices; Managed Care Settings; Home Health Care; Skilled Nursing Facilities	
New Hampshire	X	X	PENDING	Hospitals, Long Term Care facilities, Inpatient or Outpatient hospice settings, Ambulatory Care Clinics	NH H 115 Chapter No. 164

[1] Not addressed in laws or regulations but may do so if acting as an agent of the prescriber. *National Association of Boards of Pharmacy 2006 Survey* results.

[2] Subject to interpretation. Not specifically addressed in law or regulation. However, on June 2, 2000, the Iowa Board of Pharmacy Examiners issued a Declaratory Order specific to whether or not pharmaceutical case management (as defined in the relative Medicaid waiver) was within Iowa pharmacists' scope of practice. The Board ruled that, "PCM services that are delivered in the manner described in the Petition to fall within the scope of the practice of pharmacy in the State of Iowa. However, the Iowa Board of Pharmacy responded to the *National Association of Boards of Pharmacy's 2006 Survey* that there is not collaborative drug therapy authority in the State of Iowa

[3] Medical Practice Act interpreted to permit delegation to pharmacist.

[4] Michigan's Medical Practice Act is interpreted to permit delegation to a pharmacist.

continued on next page

Table 1. CDTM Comparison Chart by State (cont'd)

STATE	CDTM	STATUTE	REGULATION	PRACTICE SETTING	2005-2006 ACTIVITY
New Jersey	X	X		All	
New Mexico	X	X		All	
New York		PENDING			
North Carolina	X	X	X	All	
North Dakota	X	X	X	Institutional Settings: Hospitals; Skilled Nursing Facilities; Swing Bed Facilities; Clinics	
Ohio	X	X	X	All	
Oklahoma					
Oregon	X		X	All	
Pennsylvania	X	X	X	Institutional Settings	
Rhode Island	X	X		Hospital (including outpatient clinics), Nursing Homes	
South Carolina[5]	X	X		All	
South Dakota	X	X		All	
Tennessee[6]	X			All	
Texas	X	X	X	All	
Utah	X	X		All	
Vermont	X		X	Institutional Settings	
Virginia	X	X	X	All	
Washington	X	X	X	All	
West Virginia	X	X		Institutional Settings & 5 Pilot Sites in Community Settings	Act No. 184 2005
Wisconsin[7]	X	X		All	
Wyoming	X	X	X	All	
Total:	43				
Pending:	4				

[5] Subject to interpretation. The South Carolina's Board of Pharmacy responded to the *National Association of Boards of Pharmacy's 2006 Survey* that there isn't collaborative drug therapy authority in the State of South Carolina. However, several definitions in the practice act suggest otherwise: "practice of pharmacy means…drug administration…provision of those acts or services necessary to provide pharmacy care and drug therapy management; "drug therapy management is that practice of pharmacy which involves the expertise of the pharmacist in a collaborative effort with the practitioner and other health care providers to ensure the highest quality health care services; and "prescription drug orders means a lawful order from a practitioner …and including orders derived from collaborative pharmacy practice."

[6] Tennessee Board of Pharmacy responded to the *National Association of Boards of Pharmacy's 2006 Survey* that there is collaborative drug therapy authority in the State of Tennessee. However, it is not specifically cited in law. "Pharmaceutical Care is defined as including, "developing relationships with licensed practitioners to enable the pharmacist to accomplish comprehensive management of a patient's pharmacy related care and to enhance a patient's wellness, quality of life and optimize outcomes; and communicating to the health care provider any knowledge of unexpected or adverse response to drug therapy, or resolving unexpected or adverse response; and having a pharmacist accessible at all time to patients and healthcare providers to respond to their questions and needs."

[7] Medical Practice Act interpreted to permit delegation to pharmacist.

- Difficulty obtaining physician acceptance
- Lack of support from administration
- Slow process for getting credentialing status
- Inadequate knowledge of billing and clinical skills
- Indifferent attitude of pharmacy practitioners
- Lack of cohesive vision for practice models
- Insufficient space to perform services
- Outcomes failing to meet expectations[4]

CDTM CHART

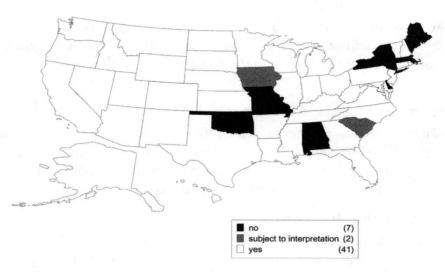

■ no	(7)
■ subject to interpretation	(2)
□ yes	(41)

Figure 1. CDTM Map

Essential elements for a pharmacist to be effective in providing CDTM include:

- A collaborative practice environment where physicians and pharmacists share responsibility for the patient
- Direct interaction with patients
- Access to medical records, which includes history, assessments, and laboratory and procedure results
- A requisite level of education, training, knowledge, skills, and ability
- Timely and appropriate documentation of activities
- Mechanisms to measure and ensure quality patient care
- Payment for pharmacists' services[2]

Process for Starting a CDTM Service

Eight steps should be followed for establishing a CDTM service:

1. Perform a needs assessment
2. Develop the program
3. Allocate resources
4. Market CDTM services
5. Identify at-risk patients

6. Provide the service
7. Determine outcomes of the service
8. Improve the service[5]

At every step, relationships with physicians and payers must be fostered. Physicians should understand that the pharmacists' activities are collaborative in nature and do not usurp their authority, but rather enhance the level of care provided to patients.[5]

Performing a Needs Assessment

Performing a needs assessment will identify a patient population that could benefit from CDTM services. Discussing unmet health care needs with stakeholders may assist in narrowing the focus; stakeholders include administrators, physicians, third-party payers, and potential patients.

Developing the Program

The goals and elements of the CDTM program should be predetermined. Logistics must be deliberated; they include pharmacist responsibilities, length of patient appointments or group classes, frequency of visits, and the method of intervention documentation and communication to the referring provider.

Allocating Resources

Consideration must be given to the allocation of resources, including pharmacist salaries, pharmacist credentialing, number and length of appointments, adequate space to see patients, and where the service will be offered (e.g., physicians' offices, hospitals, free clinics, community pharmacies, and long-term care facilities).

Marketing CDTM Services

Services can be marketed to health systems, physicians, and payers by inquiring about their health care needs and explaining how pharmacists can assist in meeting those needs. Advertising to patients may include posting flyers, mailing newsletters, and placing leaflets with prescriptions.

Identifying At-Risk Patients

Identifying prospective patients can occur in many ways such as using billing codes or prescription databases, self- and physician referrals, and proactively screening patients.

Providing the Service

When planning is complete, the program can begin accepting referrals and seeing patients. National clinical guidelines provide an outline of assessments to conduct and education to provide at each visit. Initial visits are longer than follow-up visits. A 45- to 60-minute appointment typically allows enough time to explain the purpose of the visit, gather information about patient history, complete a basic physical assessment, and determine and discuss the therapeutic plan. The length of return visits is determined by patient complexity and the educational topics to be covered and may range from 10 to 45 minutes.

Determining Outcomes

The outcomes to be measured should be determined prior to initiation of the service so that appropriate data are collected along the way. Outcome measures may include clinical parameters, quality of life, patient and provider satisfaction, and pharmacoeconomic analyses. Identifying areas for improvement and developing solutions to encountered problems will assist in improving the program.

Improving the Service

Once outcomes are collected, areas for improvement should be identified and strategies for improving should be developed and implemented. If program goals have been met, consider expanding the program to address other needs or a larger patient population.

Harborview Medical Center (HMC) Experience

Over 20 years ago, the HMC Pharmacy department began to develop clinical pharmacy services in the ambulatory care clinics. We started by sending a pharmacist with a medication cart and a typewriter to the Asthma Clinic that met one afternoon per week. The pharmacist dispensed asthma medications, provided intensive patient education, and consulted with the physicians on medication-related issues in clinic. The pharmacist developed therapeutic guidelines in collaboration with the physicians and within a short time were starting, adjusting, and discontinuing asthma medications. These physicians talked with their colleagues and, before long, we were being asked to send pharmacists to several of our clinics. Due to resource limitations, we prioritized these requests for special patient populations with unique needs who could benefit the most from a decentralized pharmacy care model. Over the next few years, we provided pharmacists to our Geriatric Clinic, International Medicine Clinic (internal medicine clinic for non-English speaking patients), Pediatric Clinic, and HIV/AIDS Clinic.

Ultimately, our largest adult primary care clinic asked our department to participate in a quality improvement initiative around the care of hypertensive patients. There were three teams of providers in the clinic. One team provided usual care to their hypertensive patients; the second team received education from the clinical pharmacist regarding hypertension management; and the third team referred their hypertensive patients to the clinical pharmacist for medication management. The patients on the third team demonstrated improved blood pressure control, improved adherence to medications, and reduced medication and overall health care costs. After seeing these results, our Chief Operating Officer asked if the clinical pharmacist could help improve the care of patients with other chronic conditions and approved a permanent pharmacist position in the clinic. Our services grew from there, and we now have pharmacists in all of our primary care and most of our specialty clinics.

In addition, we participate on several interdisciplinary care teams to improve quality and efficiency of care. This helps integrate pharmacists into the standard patient care model at HMC. For example, we sent an interdisciplinary team to a statewide Diabetes Collaborative to improve care for patients with diabetes. Based on available evidence, this team established an ideal care model for patients with diabetes and defined roles for each caregiver to optimize care for these patients.

The continued success of our program depends in part on maintaining highly competent staff and accessible, trained management. The necessary qualifications for our clinical pharmacy specialist positions include a Doctor of Pharmacy degree; 2 years of residency training with the second post-graduate year (PGY2) in primary care, family medicine, or geriatrics; and board certification in Pharmacotherapy by the Board of Pharmaceutical Specialties (BPS). Continuing proficiency is assessed annually with evaluations from physicians and fellow pharmacists.

The professional development of management includes obtaining an advanced degree such as a Masters in Health Administration (MHA) and routine participation in leadership development programs. Managers maintain accessibility by keeping their doors open to employees, routinely visiting team members in clinics, and participating in monthly clinical staff meetings. In addition they mentor staff members to lead various projects, which facilitates increased leadership skills among the clinical pharmacy specialists.

An important aspect of implementing our CDTM program included developing a vision statement, service goals, and standards of care (as follows).

Ambulatory Pharmacy Services Vision Statement
Set the national standard for the provision of care. Achieve recognition as leaders in providing fully integrated, patient-centered, pharmaceutical care through innovative, safe, cost-effective, and accessible pharmacy services. Provide excellence in research and training.

Ambulatory Pharmacy Services Goals
Service and Program Excellence
- Optimize adherence of medication regimen
- Provide patient care and education within an interdisciplinary care framework

- Optimize disease state management utilizing evidence-based medicine
- Efficiently and consistently document patient care activities and interventions with a progress note in the patient's medical chart
- Collect and utilize pharmacy-related outcomes to improve patient care
- Develop and utilize ambulatory pharmacy standards of practice (see below)
- Enhance partnering with other members of the health care team
- Provide relevant, thoughtful, and timely drug information consultations to other health care providers
- Develop a strategy for partnering between inpatient and ambulatory pharmacists and between the distribution pharmacists and the clinic-based pharmacists
- Enhance the medication regimen evaluation for new and refill medications for safe, effective, and appropriate use
- Provide high quality, well-coordinated practicum and experiential sites for the University of Washington School of Pharmacy Pharm.D. students, University of Washington Academic Medical Center (UW Medical Center, Harborview Medical Center, and the Seattle Cancer Care Alliance) residents, and HMC interns
- Respect the professional partnership with HMC patients

Human Resources
- Invest in highly qualified staff with demonstrated professional, technical, and interpersonal competencies
- Provide on-site, relevant, high-quality continuous professional development for pharmacy staff

Financial Viability
- Manage resources in a manner that supports program needs, optimizes effectiveness and efficiency, and contributes to a sustainable contribution margin
- Partner with the patient and health care providers in making medication decisions based upon their pharmacy benefit

Administration
- Maintain an environment that promotes accessible and skilled management to oversee the Ambulatory Pharmacy program

HMC Pharmacy Patient Care Standards of Practice

Standard: A progress note shall be written at each patient visit.

Standard: The pharmacist shall ensure that the subjective and objective information is consistent with the assessment and plan within the progress note.

Standard: Past medical history, medication history, and family history shall be noted by a provider at least once for each patient.

Standard: Social, diet, and exercise history shall be recorded when appropriate.

Standard: Current prescription and non-prescription medication shall be updated and documented at each visit.

Standard: Adherence to the therapeutic plan shall be assessed at each visit.

Standard: Each patient visit shall include questioning and education concerning disease control, signs or symptoms of disease progression or new complications, and signs or symptoms of adverse reactions.

Standard: Each patient visit shall document appropriate objective information such as laboratory, physical assessment data, and vital signs, as necessary for disease state management.

Standard: All patient counseling concerning drug therapy, adherence, diet, exercise, and other lifestyle factors shall be documented and patient understanding assessed and documented.

Standard: Therapeutic goals shall be clearly stated and documented.

Standard: Appropriate recommendations and drug regimen changes shall be made and documented in the plan.

Standard: Appropriate timing of follow-up visit shall be included in every plan.

Standard: The pharmacist shall follow the HMC guidelines for suspending a relationship with a patient who fails to keep appointments. The referring provider shall be notified for further follow-up.

Standard: Data collection assessing outcomes will be integrated into clinical guidelines and data collection performed by pharmaceutical care pharmacists.

Standard: Nationally recognized treatment guidelines and clinic-specific standards of practice shall be utilized for the chronic and acute illnesses, which clinic-based pharmacists manage.

About This Book

The majority of this handbook contains guidelines for CDTM of multiple therapeutic areas. These topics were chosen because they are disease states commonly managed by pharmacists as well as the areas of CDTM practice at our institution. The guidelines are not intended to serve as exhaustive therapeutic resources, but rather to provide a framework for providing CDTM services.

Case studies contained in several of the chapters serve to demonstrate the application of the guidelines in a patient care scenario.

As mentioned above, a key component of CDTM is assessing outcomes and improving the service. The chapter on pharmacy outcomes provides information on various approaches to collecting quality data and methods for assessing the data, as well as intervention tracking systems used to evaluate and demonstrate the value of clinical pharmacist services. The chapter on privileging and credentialing details the process used for ensuring clinical pharmacy specialists have the necessary education, training, knowledge, skills, and ability to successfully provide CDTM services.

Summary

Primary care clinics offer opportunities for pharmacists to work in partnership with patients and health providers to direct cost-effective therapies and manage both the individual patient and large populations. Pharmacists through collaborative agreements can effectively improve patient outcomes by providing evidence-based pharmacotherapeutic consultation and direct patient management. Motivational interviewing skills assist in identifying a patient's barriers to adherence (medication and lifestyle), problem solving, and developing patient-specific goals that will achieve health care objectives and improve outcomes. Continuous communication; face-to-face encounters; working side-by-side with patients and providers to develop a common message and plan; sharing of patient information and progress; and collaborative efforts with providers have allowed our clinical pharmacy services to grow and evolve. Today, clinical pharmacy services are an integral part of daily patient care at our institution. We hope the information in this handbook will help others develop, implement, and expand their clinical pharmacy services through CDTM.

References

1. Carmichael JM, O'Connell MB, Devine B, et al. Collaborative drug therapy management by pharmacists. *Pharmacotherapy*. 1997; 17(5):1050–61.

2. Hammond RW, Schwartz AH, Campbell MJ, et al. Collaborative drug therapy management by pharmacists—2003. *Pharmacotherapy*. 2003; 23(9):1210–25.

3. American Society of Health-System Pharmacists. Issue paper: collaborative drug therapy management. Available at http://www.ashp.org/s_ashp/docs/files/ GAD_CDTM_issuePaper.pdf. Accessed February 27, 2007.

4. Singla D. MTM services: opportunities for collaborative practice relationships. Available at http://www.pharmacytimes.com/article.cfm?ID=2003. Accessed March 18, 2007.

5. Scott MA, Fritsch M, Powell LK, et al. Collaborative drug therapy management. Available at http://secure.pharmacytimes.com/lessons/200112-01.asp. Accessed March 14, 2007.

Treatment Guidelines/Example Protocols

Coronary Artery Disease

Carrie L. Yuan

Coronary artery disease (CAD) is the most common type of heart disease in the Western world. Alternatively known as coronary heart disease (CHD), ischemic heart disease, and atherosclerotic heart disease, CAD affects approximately 15.8 million Americans.[1] It is the leading cause of death in the United States.[2] Pharmacists, especially in collaborative practices, have numerous opportunities to assist with the prevention and treatment of CAD.

Indications

Identification of Patients with CAD/Atherosclerotic Disease

1. Patients with prior history or diagnosis of unstable angina, non-ST elevation myocardial infarction (NSTEMI), or acute MI (ST-elevation MI).
2. Patients with chronic stable angina, including those who were previously symptomatic prior to percutaneous coronary intervention (PCI) or coronary artery bypass grafting (CABG).
3. Patients with peripheral or cerebral vascular disease with or without history of ischemic stroke.
4. Patients with diabetes or multiple risk factors that confer a 10-year cardiovascular event risk of >20% are considered to have CAD-equivalent risk.[3]

Management

Pharmacotherapy to Reduce Mortality

1. *Antiplatelet medications.* Daily aspirin therapy (81–325 mg) is recommended in

15

the absence of contraindications. When aspirin is absolutely contraindicated, clopidogrel 75 mg daily is the preferred alternative. Ticlopidine is a third antiplatelet option but carries the risk of neutropenia and lacks sufficient evidence to show decreased adverse cardiovascular events.[4]

2. *Beta blockers.* Unless contraindicated, beta blocker therapy is initiated or continued in all patients with a history of MI, acute coronary syndrome, or left ventricular dysfunction with or without heart failure symptoms. This is in accordance with the American Heart Association (AHA)/American College of Cardiology (ACC) Guidelines for Secondary Prevention for Patients with Coronary and Other Atherosclerotic Vascular Disease.[5]

3. *Lipid-lowering agents.* All patients with known CAD are treated with a HMG CoA reductase inhibitor (statin) to reduce LDL-C, the primary target in lipid therapy.[5,6] If the LDL-C goal is not achieved with statin monotherapy, consider adding a second agent such as ezetimibe, fibrates, cholesterol-binding resins, or niacin. Selection of the second agent is influenced by concomitant drug therapy, secondary lipoprotein goals, patient drug history, metabolic parameters, and cost.

4. *Renin–angiotensin–aldosterone system inhibitors.* Unless contraindicated, angiotensin-converting enzyme (ACE) inhibitors are initiated or continued in all patients status post-MI or with decreased left ventricular function (ejection fraction of <40%).[5] Strongly consider initiating an ACE inhibitor in all other patients with CAD/atherosclerotic disease, especially those with diabetes, chronic kidney disease, or hypertension. Patients who are intolerant of ACE inhibitors may be given an angiotensin receptor blocker (ARB).

Pharmacotherapy to Improve Symptoms

1. *Nitrates/beta blockers.* Beta blockers improve anginal symptoms and reduce the risk of adverse cardiovascular events in patients with chronic stable angina.[4,7] Nitrates provide symptomatic relief of anginal symptoms; however, they have not been shown to decrease mortality. A combination of beta blockers and nitrates will often attenuate the reflex tachycardia that may occur with nitrate monotherapy. It is important to provide patients with comprehensive education on appropriate use of immediate-acting nitrates for relief of acute anginal symptoms.

2. *Calcium antagonists.* Slow-release and long-acting calcium antagonists are effective for relieving symptoms in patients with chronic stable angina.[4] Calcium antagonists are often used in patients who are intolerant to beta blockers or in combination with beta blockers when the maximal tolerable beta blocker dose does not adequately control anginal symptoms. Like nitrates, the calcium antagonists provide symptomatic relief of anginal symptoms but have not been shown to decrease mortality. Avoid using immediate-release calcium antagonists due to the increased risk of adverse cardiovascular events.

Management of Risk Factors

1. *Hypertension.* High blood pressure must be treated as a means of reducing the risk of adverse cardiovascular events. The Seventh Report of the Joint National Committee on Prevention, Detection, Evaluation, and Treatment of High Blood Pressure (JNC 7)[8] describes compelling indications for the use of specific antihypertensive drugs.

2. *Tobacco cessation.* All tobacco users should be advised of the health risks of continued use (provide a strong quit message) and offered intensive smoking cessation counseling. Continually assess readiness to quit at each visit for those continuing to use tobacco.

3. *Physical activity.* All patients should be counseled to gradually increase their aerobic activity level as tolerated to a target of 30 minutes daily.

4. *Nutrition.* Although dietary intervention alone has not been shown to be beneficial, it may be valuable when used in combination with exercise and cholesterol-lowering medications in patients with CAD. It is important to provide basic dietary education and refer patients who may benefit from more intensive education or consultation with a registered dietician.

Goals of Therapy

1. *Lipids.* Treat to achieve a target LDL-C of <100 mg/dL in all patients with known CAD or CAD risk-equivalent.[6] In very high-risk patients, or in those with baseline LDL-C of <100 mg/dL, it may be appropriate to opt for a lower LDL-C target of <70 mg/dL.[9] In moderate- to high-risk patients with low baseline LDL-C, aim to achieve at least 30–40% reduction in baseline LDL-C.[10] In secondary prevention of coronary events, aggressively titrate statin doses to achieve the LDL-C target. Refer to Chapter 2 for discussion of lipid-lowering drugs and monitoring parameters.

2. *Antianginal therapy.* Titrate antianginal therapy to minimize the occurrence of anginal symptoms. Track frequency of use of "as needed" nitroglycerin as one marker of symptom control. For patients on beta blockers, titrate the dose according to symptom control, maximum tolerated dose, or a maximal dose that achieves a resting heart rate of 50 to 60 beats per minute.

3. *Hypertension.* Treat blood pressure to achieve a goal of <140/90 mm Hg, or <130/80 mm Hg in patients with diabetes or chronic kidney disease, according to JNC 7 guidelines.[8] Refer to Chapter 3 for discussion of specific antihypertensive drugs and monitoring parameters.

Clinical Pharmacy Goals

1. Identify patients with documented CAD or at risk for atherothrombotic events (peripheral or cerebral atherosclerotic disease, diabetes, presence of multiple risk factors).

2. Ensure that appropriate drug therapies are initiated and continued to modify the underlying atherosclerotic process and prevent recurrent events.

3. Educate patients regarding their disease state, therapeutic lifestyle changes, and the general use and importance of drug therapies. Guide patients towards increased self-management of their condition.

Outcome Measures

1. Process measures: Unless contraindicated, all patients with documented CAD or its equivalent will receive disease-modifying therapies, including acetylsalicylic acid (ASA), beta blockers, ACE inhibitors, lipid-lowering therapies, smoking cessation counseling, and diet and exercise counseling.

2. Surrogate clinical markers: Lipid and blood pressure goals achieved.

3. Health outcome measures: Reduction in secondary cardiovascular, cerebral, and peripheral ischemic events.

Patient Information Resources

1. National Heart, Lung, Blood Institute website on CAD: http://www.nhlbi.nih.gov/health/dci/Diseases/Cad/CAD_WhatIs.html

2. American Heart Association: http://www.americanheart.org

CASE STUDY

S: Ms. J is a 53 yo female s/p NSTEMI 2 months ago. Catheterization demonstrated 50% mid-LAD lesion and a 95% second obtuse lesion that was stented with subsequent 0% residual stenosis. Ms. J reports that she is slowly recovering her functional status. For the most part, she has not had any chest pain during her activities of daily living, although she has had two brief episodes of chest pain since discharge. The first episode occurred while she was walking up stairs at a moderate pace. She experienced a few seconds of chest pain, which resolved with rest. The second episode occurred this morning when she developed a few minutes of chest pain after showering and dressing. This again resolved with rest.

Allergies: NKDA

Current medications:

Atorvastatin 10 mg daily since hospital discharge

Metoprolol 12.5 mg BID

Lisinopril 10 mg BID

Clopidogrel 75 mg daily

ASA EC 81 mg daily

Multivitamin daily

O: Vital signs: BP 114/56, HR 72

Lipids: TC 222, TG 165, LDL 139, HDL 50

A/P: S/p recent NSTEMI with two brief episodes of exertional chest pain. *This patient has inadequate control of angina symptoms. She is receiving all recommended drug therapy to decrease mortality.*

1. Increase metoprolol to 25 mg BID. *Increasing the dose of the beta blocker should improve her symptoms. There is room for upward titration of her metoprolol since her resting heart rate is 72, which is well above the dose-limiting HR of 50–60.*

2. Prescribe sublingual nitroglycerin prn chest pain and educate pt on when to seek emergency care for ongoing angina. *She should have a prescription for "as needed" nitroglycerin for relief of anginal symptoms.*

3. Increase atorvastatin to 20 mg daily. Plan to recheck lipids in 6–8 weeks. *She has been on the current dose of atorvastatin for 2 months and has not achieved her LDL target of 100 mg/dL. Therefore, a dosage increase is warranted.*

4. Follow-up with cardiology clinic as scheduled in 2 weeks; return to clinic with PCP in 4 weeks.

5. Monitor prn nitroglycerin use and consider further titrating metoprolol dose if anginal symptoms continue. *If anginal symptoms continue on the maximum dose of metoprolol, options include adding a calcium channel blocker or a long-acting nitrate.*

References

1. Rosamond W, Flegel K, Friday G, et al. Heart disease and stroke statistics—2007 update: a report from the American Heart Association Statistics Committee and Stroke Statistics Subcommittee. *Circulation*. 2007; 115:e69–171.

2. Heron MP, Smith BL. Deaths: leading causes for 2003. *Natl Vital Stat Rep*. 2007; 55:1–92.

3. National Institutes of Health; National Heart, Lung, and Blood Institute; National Cholesterol Education Program 10-year Risk Calculator. Available at http://www.nhlbi.nih.gov/guidelines/cholesterol/index.htm. Accessed October 23, 2006.

4. Gibbons RJ, Abrams J, Chatterjee K, et al. ACC/AHA 2002 guideline update for the management of patients with chronic stable angina: a report of the American

College of Cardiology/American Heart Association Task Force on Practice Guidelines. Available at http://www.acc.org/qualityandscience/clinical/guidelines/stable/update_index.htm. Accessed June 14, 2006.

5. Smith SC, Allen J, Blair SN, et al. AHA/ACC guidelines for secondary prevention for patients with coronary and other atherosclerotic vascular disease: 2006 update. *Circulation*. 2006; 113:2363–72.

6. Executive summary of the third report of the National Cholesterol Education Program (NCEP) Expert Panel on detection, evaluation, and treatment of high blood cholesterol in adults. *JAMA*. 2001; 285(19):2486–95.

7. Pepine CJ, Cohn PF, Deedwania PC, et al. Effects of treatment on outcome in mildly symptomatic patients with ischemia during daily life. The Atenolol Silent Ischemia Study (ASIST). *Circulation*. 1994; 90:762–8.

8. Chobanian AV, Bakris GL, Black HR, et al. The seventh report of the Joint National Committee on Prevention, Detection, Evaluation, and Treatment of High Blood Pressure (JNC 7 Report). *JAMA*. 2003; 289:2560–71.

9. Grundy SM, Cleeman JI, Merz CN, et al. Implications of recent clinical trials for the National Cholesterol Education Program Adult Treatment Panel III Guidelines. *Circulation*. 2004; 110:227–39.

10. Heart Protection Study Collaborative Group. MRC/BHF Heart Protection Study of cholesterol lowering with simvastatin in 20,536 high-risk individuals: a randomised placebo-controlled trial. *Lancet*. 2002; 360:7–22.

Dyslipidemia

Alvin Goo

Cardiovascular disease (CVD) risk reduction involves managing multiple modifiable factors that include blood pressure, smoking cessation, low-density lipoprotein (LDL) cholesterol, metabolic syndrome, weight loss, exercise, and nutrition. The Third Report of the National Cholesterol Education Program (NCEP III) guidelines focus on lowering LDL based on the benefits demonstrated in multiple studies, particularly for secondary prevention of CVD.[1] It remains uncertain if the other cholesterol factors, high-density lipoprotein (HDL) and triglycerides (TG), also contribute to CVD; further research is needed.

Studies indicate LDL lowering with statins reduces cardiovascular events and mortality in patients with previous history of CVD. Studies also demonstrate a reduction in cardiovascular events, but not mortality, in high-risk patients such as type 2 diabetes mellitus without history of CVD, stroke/transient ischemic attacks (TIA), or with elevated LDL and high risk for CVD. Controversy exists whether cholesterol treatment should be focused on titration and achievement of specified LDL goals, achieving a particular percent LDL reduction, or if treatment can be simplified by determining a specific standard statin dose. Future studies must focus on the determination of the most clinically effective statin dose. This section focuses on the treatment of dyslipidemia; however, it is crucial to manage the whole patient and various modifiable cardiovascular risk factors.

Indications

Results of secondary prevention lipid-lowering trials demonstrate significant reductions in total and cardiovascular morbidity and mortality. The most significant health benefits can be achieved treating patients at greatest risk for future CHD events (e.g., established CVD, recent acute coronary syndrome, or type 2 diabetes at high risk for CVD). Identify patients at the highest risk for developing cardiovascular events through provider referral and medical database queries.

High-risk patients include, but are not limited to, those with:

1. Acute coronary syndrome (ACS)
2. Previous cardiovascular events
3. Type 2 diabetes (DM)
4. Stroke or TIA
5. Metabolic syndrome

Risk Factors

1. Age male $\geq$45, female $\geq$55 or premature menopause
2. Family history of premature coronary heart disease (CHD) or sudden death <55 in father or other male first degree relative or <65 in mother or other female first-degree relative
3. Current cigarette smoking
4. Hypertension (BP $\geq$140/90 mmHg or taking antihypertensive therapy)
5. Low high-density lipoprotein (HDL) <40 mg/dL
6. Diabetes

   Protective Factor: High HDL $\geq$60 mg/dL (presence removes one risk factor from total count)

CHD Risk Equivalents

1. Diabetes
2. Peripheral vascular disease
3. Abdominal aneurysm
4. Carotid artery disease
5. Framingham 10-year risk >20%

Table 2-1 summarizes treatment thresholds based on risk factors and baseline LDL.

Table 2-1. NCEP III LDL Cholesterol Goals

Patient Category	LDL Goal	Consider Drug Therapy
Without CHD, 0–1 risk factor	<160 mg/dL	$\geq$190 mg/dL (160–189 mg/dL LDL-lowering treatment optional)
Without CHD, $\geq$2 risk factors (10-yr risk for CHD $\leq$20%)	<130 mg/dL	10-yr risk <10%: $\geq$160 mg/dL 10-yr risk 10–20%: $\geq$130 mg/dL

continued on next page

Table 2-1. NCEP III LDL Cholesterol Goals (cont'd)

Patient Category	LDL Goal	Consider Drug Therapy
CHD, DM, or CHD risk equivalent (10-yr risk for CHD >20%)	<100 mg/dL	≥100 mg/dL (100–129 mg/dL LDL-lowering treatment optional)
Optional ACS, or DM with CHD and baseline LDL approximately 100 mg/dL	<70 mg/dL	≥70 mg/dL

Management

Patient Assessment

1. Assess patient's cardiovascular risk factors or individual characteristics.
2. Calculate the Framingham 10-year risk for cardiovascular disease. See **Tables 2-2 and 2-3** or http://hin.nhlbi.nih.gov/atpiii/calculator.asp?usertype=prof to calculate.

Table 2-2. Estimate of 10-Year Risk for Men

Framingham Point Scores by Age Group

Age	Points
20–34	-9
35–39	-4
40–44	0
45–49	3
50–54	6
55–59	8
60–64	10
65–69	11
70–74	12
75–79	13

Framingham Point Scores by Age Group and Total Cholesterol

Total Cholesterol	Age 20–39	Age 40–49	Age 50–59	Age 60–69	Age 70–79
<160	0	0	0	0	0
160–199	4	3	2	1	0
200–239	7	5	3	1	0
240–279	9	6	4	2	1
280+	11	8	5	3	1

continued on next page

Framingham Point Scores by Age and Smoking Status

	Age 20–39	Age 40–49	Age 50–59	Age 60–69	Age 70–79
Nonsmoker	0	0	0	0	0
Smoker	8	5	3	1	1

Framingham Point Scores by HDL Level

HDL	Points
60+	-1
50–59	0
40–49	1
<40	2

Framingham Point Scores by Systolic Blood Pressure and Treatment Status

Systolic BP	If Untreated	If Treated
<120	0	0
120–129	0	1
130–139	1	2
140–159	1	2
160+	2	3

10-Year Risk by Total Framingham Point Scores

Point Total	10-Year Risk
<0	<1%
0	1%
1	1%
2	1%
3	1%
4	1%
5	2%
6	2%
7	3%
8	4%
9	5%
10	6%
11	8%
12	10%
13	12%
14	16%
15	20%
16	25%
17 or more	>30%

Table 2-3. Estimate of 10-Year Risk for Women

Framingham Point Scores by Age Group

Age	Points
20–34	-7
35–39	-3
40–44	0
45–49	3
50–54	6
55–59	8
60–64	10
65–69	12
70–74	14
75–79	16

Framingham Point Scores by Age Group and Total Cholesterol

Total Cholesterol	Age 20–39	Age 40–49	Age 50–59	Age 60–69	Age 70–79
<160	0	0	0	0	0
160–199	4	3	2	1	1
200–239	8	6	4	2	1
240–279	11	8	5	3	2
280+	13	10	7	4	2

Framingham Point Scores by Age and Smoking Status

	Age 20–39	Age 40–49	Age 50–59	Age 60–69	Age 70–79
Nonsmoker	0	0	0	0	0
Smoker	9	7	4	2	1

Framingham Point Scores by HDL Level

HDL	Points
60+	-1
50–59	0
40–49	1
<40	2

Framingham Point Scores by Systolic Blood Pressure and Treatment Status

Systolic BP	If Untreated	If Treated
<120	0	0
120–129	1	3
130–139	2	4
140–159	3	5
160+	4	6

continued on next page

10-Year Risk by Total Framingham Point Scores

Point Total	10-Year Risk
<9	<1%
9	1%
10	1%
11	1%
12	1%
13	2%
14	2%
15	3%
16	4%
17	5%
18	6%
19	8%
20	11%
21	14%
22	17%
23	22%
24	27%
25 or more	≥30%

3. Evaluate and identify precautions or contraindications to statins, fibrates, and niacin.

4. Assess the patient's understanding and goals of therapy.

5. Assess the patient's barriers to lifestyle and medication adherence.

Plan

1. Develop a plan with the patient to address educational needs and barriers to adherence as well as assist with setting goals.

2. Educate and encourage participation in therapeutic lifestyle modifications for all patients with LDL above goal.

3. Determine percent reduction in LDL needed to achieve goal.

4. Select appropriate statin or other lipid-lowering agent and starting dose.

5. Determine appropriate time interval for follow-up of fasting lipid panel (FLP).

6. Develop monitoring plan for hepatitis, myositis, and rhabdomyolysis.

Lipid-Lowering Agents

1. *HMG CoA reductase inhibitors (statins).* Statins remain first-line agents in lowering LDL and reducing cardiovascular morbidity and mortality. Statins are well tolerated; however, adherence after 2 years is often suboptimal. Pharmacists should conduct patient education, assess for side effects and patient

barriers to adherence, and assist with establishing and achieving patient goals on an ongoing basis.

Choice of statin is currently based on estimating the percent LDL reduction needed to obtain the LDL goal and selecting the appropriate statin dose. However, statin doses do not have a linear relationship with percent LDL lowering; doubling the statin dose does not double the percent LDL reduction. Statin dosing would be simplified if future studies determine that a specific statin dose, rather than achieving a particular LDL goal, is beneficial in reducing cardiovascular morbidity.

Statin doses can be started at a low to moderate dose and titrated up. This allows determination of the most effective dose tailored to the patient. Drawbacks of this method are increased visits and laboratory tests and possible delay in achieving the LDL goal. An alternative method is to initiate a statin at the dose that will most likely achieve the LDL goal. This does not allow titration of the statin and may lead to increased cost; however, LDL goal can be achieved within 4–8 weeks with possibly less monitoring of FLP.

Intensity of statin therapy can also be based on primary or secondary prevention. Primary prevention does not require aggressive therapy and a mid-potent statin can be initiated and titrated to LDL goal. For patients with no prior history of a cardiovascular event, LDL lowering with statins reduces the incidence of cardiovascular events but does not decrease mortality. The cost of the statin itself is the major expense involved in treating these patients. Therefore, it is important to weigh the cost effectiveness of treatment for primary prevention. Primary prevention with statins may not be cost effective for younger men and women with few risk factors. Primary prevention becomes favorable with increasing numbers of risk factors (e.g., diastolic blood pressure >95 mmHg, HDL <35 mg/dL, smoking, history of premature cardiovascular events in first degree relative, age).

Secondary prevention can be divided into ACS or past history of CVD. ACS may require more intensive and aggressive therapy, and a moderate to high potency statin may be preferred.

The following cholesterol-lowering agents are recommended as secondary or adjunctive therapy when patients fail to tolerate statins or when additional LDL lowering is desired beyond maximum statin therapy.

2. *Bile sequestering agents (resins)*. Resins bind to bile acids in the intestine and disrupt the enterohepatic recirculation of bile acids. This increases hepatic synthesis of bile acids from cholesterol, which results in increased LDL receptors and a reduction in LDL. Resins typically reduce LDL by 15–30% and may increase TG if used as monotherapy.

3. *Niacin*. Niacin reduces the hepatic synthesis and secretion of VLDL, resulting in reduction in LDL and TG and increase in HDL. Niacin in combination with a statin can potentiate LDL lowering.

4. *Fibrates.* Fibrates increase lipoprotein lipase and the metabolism of TG. The major effect of fibrates is to lower TG with minimal lowering of LDL and minimal increase in HDL. Elevated TG is associated with an increased risk of cardiovascular disease. However, randomized trials are lacking to determine if lowering TG reduces the incidence of cardiovascular disease. Severely elevated TG >600–800 mg/dL increase the risk of pancreatitis and must be addressed with fibrates.

5. *Ezetimibe.* Ezetimibe inhibits the intestinal enzyme responsible for absorbing cholesterol in the intestine. Ezetimibe reduces LDL by 18% when used alone.[2] The combination of ezetimibe and a statin results in a significant LDL reduction. The combination of ezetimibe and fibrates can also result in significant TG reduction.

6. *Omega fatty acids.* Omega fatty acids inhibit the synthesis of TG and can reduce TG by 40–45%.[3] Active components of omega fatty acids are eicosapentaenoic acid (EPA) and docosahexaenoic acid (DHA). Daily supplementation with 1 gram omega fatty acids may reduce recurrence of cardiovascular disease in patients with recent myocardial infarction.[4]

Combination Lipid-Lowering Therapy

A statin in combination with niacin, bile sequestering agents, ezetimibe, or a fibrate will provide additional LDL lowering often allowing the use of lower doses of both agents. Benefits of combination therapy remain unstudied. Studies are ongoing to determine the benefits of combination therapy versus monotherapy with a statin in reducing cardiovascular morbidity and mortality.It is important to consider the possible impact of combination therapy on reducing patient adherence, increasing drug interactions and side effects, and increasing patient cost.

HDL Therapy

Current lipid-lowering agents have minimal impact on increasing HDL. However, small increases in HDL may result in significant benefit in high-risk populations. Niacin may increase HDL to a greater extent compared to fibrates. Currently, only fibrates have been studied to determine the benefit of increasing HDL. The VA-HIT study examined the effect of gemfibrozil in groups of men with a history of cardiovascular disease, low HDL, and normal LDL. Use of gemfibrozil resulted in a small increase in HDL and significant reduction in combined cardiovascular events.[5]

Triglyceride Therapy

Fibrates and niacin reduce TG effectively. Fibrates lower TG levels to a slightly greater extent compared to niacin. Fibrates are the first-line agents when addressing moderately to severely elevated TG. Fenofibrate is an alternative if a patient is intolerant to gemfibrozil. Omega fatty acids, flax seed oil alone or in addition to fibrates, and niacin may also be beneficial in lowering severely elevated TG levels. Statins combined with fibrates or niacin are associated with increased hepatitis and myositis; however, this combination is very beneficial especially in patients with diabetes or mixed dyslipidemia (elevated LDL and TG and low HDL). The combination of statins with either fibrates or niacin requires ongoing assessment for symptoms of hepatitis or myositis.

Dosing Guidelines

1. For primary prevention and CHD risk equivalent requiring <35% reduction in LDL, utilize generic lovastatin, pravastatin, or simvastatin.
2. For secondary prevention, CHD risk equivalent requiring >35% reduction in LDL, ACS, or situations requiring rapid reduction in LDL, utilize higher potency statins atorvastatin, rosuvastatin, or simvastatin.
3. Initiation doses:
    a. Initiate dose based on percent LDL reduction required (may be most appropriate for secondary prevention).
    b. Patient response will vary and is difficult to predict.

Monitoring

1. Fasting lipid panel (FLP) no sooner than 6–8 weeks after starting therapy or dose increase.
2. Liver function tests (LFTs) with FLP or 6–8 weeks after dose increase and periodically thereafter. Discontinue lipid therapy if LFTs remain persistently elevated 3 times the upper limit of normal (see **Table 2-4**). Statin-induced hepatoxicity is rare. There is little evidence that asymptomatic isolated increases in LFTs lead to hepatotoxicity. Monitoring for elevation of bilirubin in the presence of elevated liver aminotransferase levels may indicate hepatotoxicity and should be considered. The National Lipid Association Statin Safety Task Force suggests regular monitoring of liver function enzymes is not beneficial in reducing the incidence of statin-induced hepatotoxicity.[6] Therefore, monitoring for clinical symptoms of hepatotoxicity is important and should be assessed on a regular basis. Symptoms include, but are not limited to, prolonged flu-like symptoms, fatigue, malaise, and jaundice.

Table 2-4. Management of Isolated Elevated Liver Transaminases

Increase in LFTs	Initial Action	Follow-Up
1–3 times upper limit of normal	Continue agent and repeat LFT in 2–4 weeks	If LFTs continue to rise, then discontinue
3–5 times upper limit of normal	Continue agent and repeat LFT with bilirubin within 1 week	If LFTs decrease to ≤3 times upper limit of normal, then continue current dose and recheck LFTs periodically. If LFTs continue to rise, hold statin and recheck

continued on next page

Table 2-4. Management of Isolated Elevated Liver Transaminases (cont'd)

Increase in LFTs	Initial Action	Follow-Up
≥5 times upper limit of normal	Hold agent and repeat LFT with bilirubin	If LFTs decrease to ≤3 times upper limit of normal, then restart statin at a lower dose and recheck LFTs

3. Development of rhabdomyolysis is rare. However, myositis can occur and patients should be assessed for symptoms of muscle aches/discomfort, soreness, weakness, or cramps.

4. Monitor for symptoms of myositis and hepatitis, particularly with combination therapy or presence of renal insufficiency.

5. Check CPK or LFTs with symptoms of myositis or hepatitis.

Follow-Up Visit Activities

1. Educate patient regarding medication(s) and lifestyle modification (nutrition, exercise, smoking, alcohol)

2. Assess barriers to adherence

3. Assess history of CVD and CVD risk factors

4. Assess for signs and symptoms of CVD (SOB, CP, fatigue, weakness, HR, BP)

5. Assess for side effects or intolerance
    a. Hepatitis: Prolonged flu-like symptoms, malaise, jaundice
    b. Myositis: Muscle aches/discomfort, weakness, fever, abdominal discomfort

6. Assess for drug interactions

7. If at goal, continue statin therapy and recheck FLP in 1 year

8. If not at goal, then increase statin and recheck FLP in 6–8 weeks

9. If not at goal and at maximum high-dose statin, then evaluate LDL reduction achieved:
    a. If achieved LDL reduction of 30–40%, then continue same dose (particularly primary prevention or low-risk type 2 diabetes).
    b. If 30–40% reduction not achieved, consider addition of ezetimibe, niacin, or resin.
    c. Achieving a 50% reduction in LDL is difficult to reach. If clinically appropriate, then consider moderate dose of high potency statin in combination with ezetimibe, niacin, or resin.

Goals of Therapy

LDL Goals

Table 2-1 lists LDL goals for various risk groups. **Table 2-5** further delineates LDL goals for patients with CHD and CHD risk equivalents.

Table 2-5. LDL Goals for Patients with CHD and CHD Equivalents

Baseline LDL	Goal LDL
≥130 mg/dL	<100 mg/dL or reduction of at least 30–40%
100–129 mg/dL	<100 mg/dL or reduction of at least 30–40%
Near 100 mg/dL	Reduction of at least 30–40%
<100 mg/dL	Optional <70 mg/dL or reduction of at least 30–40%

The 2004 update to the NCEP guidelines added an additional optional LDL goal of <70 mg/dL in very high-risk patients.[7] This goal is for very high-risk patients with baseline LDL around 100 mg/dL. Aim to achieve LDL lowering of at least 30–40%.[7] The PROVE-It trial suggests lowering LDL <70 mg/dL reduces events immediately post MI.[8] However, it is important to take into account the baseline characteristics of the study. The patients randomized recently experienced ACS and mean baseline LDL was 106 mg/dL. It is unknown if the measured LDL corresponded with patients' actual LDL values because they were measured after the ACS event, which may have falsely lowered the LDL. Nonetheless, it is important to recognize the LDL goal of <70 mg/dL applies to patients with recent ACS and baseline LDL near 110 mg/dL. The benefit of lowering LDL <70 mg/dL when the initial LDL is >160 mg/dL after ACS—although theoretically logical and proposed by many—is uncertain and requires further investigation and verification.

Additional Goals

1. Achieving LDL goal is the primary focus of therapy
2. Total cholesterol <200 mg/dL
3. TG <150 mg/dL
4. Non-HDL cholesterol (total – HDL) 30 mg/dL higher than LDL goal (e.g., if LDL goal <100 mg/dL, then non-HDL goal <130 mg/dL)
5. Address low HDL <40 mg/dL
6. Decrease cardiovascular morbidity and mortality

Clinical Pharmacy Goals

1. Identify and obtain cholesterol levels for patients with known cardiovascular disease, CHD risk equivalent, diabetes, or with two or more risk factors.

2. Ensure patients with known cardiovascular disease, CHD risk equivalent, diabetes, or with two or more cardiovascular risk factors achieve the recommended cholesterol target goals.

3. Achieve cholesterol target goals for primary and secondary prevention in a cost-effective manner.

4. Monitor for and reduce the incidence of side effects, especially statin-induced myopathy and hepatitis.

5. Identify and address medication adherence issues.

Outcome Measures

1. Process measures: Achieve lipid goals utilizing the most cost-effective regimen.

2. Surrogate clinical markers: Achieve lipid goals based on patient's defined risk category.

3. Health outcome measures: Reduce morbidity and mortality from cardiovascular events.

Patient Information Resources

1. National Cholesterol Education Program, Information for patients: http://www.nhlbi.nih.gov/guidelines/cholesterol/index.htm

CASE STUDY

S: 58 yo male with recent MI 1 month ago presents for f/u. The provider requests your recommendation for a lipid-lowering regimen. Hx of HTN, generalized anxiety, GERD, gout.

Current medications:

  Metoprolol XL 100 mg q day

  Lisinopril 20 mg q day

  Fluoxetine 20 mg q day

  Pantoprazole 40 mg q day

O: Baseline LDL prior to MI 120 mg/dL

BP 128/80 HR 78

A/P: Dyslipidemia – LDL above goal <100 mg/dL (or possibly <70 mg/dL) for pt with CHD (s/p MI).

  1. Review nutrition and lifestyle and assist in developing patient goals.

Assess for obvious changes in nutrition, cholesterol, caloric, and sodium intake. Educate pt on necessary therapeutic lifestyle modifications.

2. Initiate simvastatin 20 mg and recheck FLP and LFT in 6 weeks, increase dose to achieve >30% LDL reduction, or LDL <70 mg/dL. *An option is to initiate low dose and gradually increase until LDL goal of <70 mg/dL or 30% reduction in LDL is achieved or to initiate at a therapeutic dose that will achieve the specific goal. Due to recent cardiac event, it is reasonable to initiate statin at a more aggressive dose. Initiate lovastatin 40 mg, pravastatin 40 mg, simvastatin 20–40 mg, atorvastatin 20–40 mg, or rosuvastatin 5– 10 mg. LDL goal is <70 mg/dL or an equivalent statin dose of atorvastatin 40–80 mg daily.*

References

1. Third Report of the National Cholesterol Education Panel (NCEP) Expert Panel on Detection, Evaluation, and Treatment of High Blood Cholesterol in Adults (Adult Treatment Panel III). *JAMA.* 2001; 285:2486–97.

2. Bays HE, Moore PB, Dreobl MA, et al. Effectiveness and tolerability of ezetimibe in patients with primary hypercholesterolemia: pooled analysis of two phase II studies. *Clin Therapeutics.* 2001; 23:1209–30.

3. Stalenhoef AF, et al. Atherosclerosis. 2000; 153:129.

4. GISSI-Prevenizone Investigators. Dietary supplementation with n-3 polyunsaturated fatty acids and vitamine E after myocardial infarction: results of the GISSI-Prevenzione trial. *Lancet.* 1999; 354:447–55.

5. Rubins H, Robins SJ, Collins D, et al. Gemfibrozil for the secondary prevention of coronary heart disease in men with low levels of high-density lipoprotein cholesterol. *N Engl J Med.* 1999; 341:410–8.

6. McKenney J. The report of the national lipid association statin safety task force. *Am J Cardiol.* 2006; 97:supplement.

7. Grundy SM, Cleeman JI, Bairey Merz CN, et al. Implications of recent clinical trials for the National Cholesterol Education Program Adult Treatment Panel III Guidelines. *Circulation.* 2004; 110:227–39.

8. Cannon CP, Braunwald E, McCabe CH, et al. Intensive versus moderate lipid lowering with statins after acute coronary syndromes. *N Engl Med.* 2004; 350:1495–504.

Bibliography

1. Downs JR, Clearfield M, Weis S, et al. Primary prevention of acute coronary events with lovastatin in men and women with average cholesterol levels: results of the AFCAPS/TexCAPS. *JAMA.* 1998; 279:1615–22.

2. Shepherd J, Cobbe SM, Ford I, et al. Prevention of coronary heart disease with pravastatin in men with hypercholesterolemia. *N Engl J Med*. 1995; 333(20):1301–7.

3. Heart Protection Study Collaborative Group. MRC/BHF heart protection study of cholesterol lowering with simvastatin in 20,536 high risk individuals; a randomized placebo-controlled trial. *Lancet*. 2002; 360:7–22.

4. Scandinavian Simvastatin Survival Study Group. Randomized trial of cholesterol-lowering in 4444 patients with coronary heart disease; the Scandinavian Simvastatin Survival Study (4S). *Lancet*. 1994; 344:1383–9.

5. The Long-Term Intervention with Pravastatin in Ischemic Disease (LIPID) Study Group. Prevention of cardiovascular events and death with pravastatin in patients with coronary heart disease and broad range of initial cholesterol levels. *N Engl J Med*. 1998; 339(19):1349–57.

6. Pedersen TR, Faergeman O, Kastelein J, et al. High-dose atorvastatin vs usual dose simvastatin for secondary prevention after myocardial infarction. The IDEAL study: a randomized controlled trial. *JAMA*. 2005; 294:2437–45.

7. LaRosa JC, Grundy SM, Waters DD, et al. Intensive lipid lowering with atorvastatin in patients with stable coronary disease. *N Engl J Med*. 2005; 352:1425–35.

8. de Lemos JA, Blazing MA, Wiviott SD, et al. Early intensive vs delayed conservative simvastatin strategy in patients with acute coronary syndrome. Phase Z of the A to Z trial. *JAMA*. 2004; 292:1307–16.

9. Colhoun HM, Betteridge DJ, Durrington PN, et al. Primary prevention of cardiovascular disease with atorvastatin in type 2 diabetes in the Collaborative Atorvastatin in Diabetes Study (CARDS): multicenter randomised placebo-controlled trial. *Lancet*. 2004; 364:685–96.

10. The Stroke Prevention by Aggressive Reduction in Cholesterol Levels (SPARCL) Investigators. High dose atorvastatin after stroke or tranisient ischemic attack. *N Engl J Med*. 2006; 355:549–59.

11. FIELD study investigators. Effects of long-term fenofibrate therapy on cardiovascular events in 9795 people with type 2 diabetes mellitus (the FIELD study): randomized control trial. *Lancet*. 2005; 366:49–61.

Hypertension

Alvin Goo

CHAPTER
3

Hypertension (HTN) affects approximately 50 million individuals in the United States and 1 billion worldwide. Unless broad and effective preventive measures are implemented, the prevalence of hypertension will continue to increase.[1] Hypertension is a major modifiable risk factor for cardiovascular disease (CVD). Current trends indicate hypertension is often undertreated and associated with poor medication and lifestyle adherence. Pharmacists play an important role then in providing patient education, identifying barriers to medication adherence, and assisting the patient in developing plans to address and improve adherence.

Numerous antihypertensive agents are available and should be tailored to address specific patient characteristics. The pharmacist's knowledge of evidence-based primary literature, pharmacokinetics, and when a particular class of antihypertensive agent provides greater benefit plays an important role in the recommendation and selection of appropriate cost-effective antihypertensive agents. The following treatment guidelines are adapted from the Seventh Report of the Joint National Committee on the Diagnosis, Evaluation, and Treatment of Hypertension for Classifying and Defining Blood Pressure levels for Adults (18 years and older).[1] For additional information, please see http://www.nhlbi.nih.gov/guidelines/hypertension.

Indications[1]

1. Adult patients ≥18 years old at high risk for developing cardiovascular events who have been referred by their primary care provider or identified from medical databases. High-risk patients include, but are not limited to, pa-

tients with diabetes, renal disease, heart failure (HF), and those with previous cardiovascular events.

2. At least two measurements are obtained on two separate visits with systolic blood pressure (SBP) >140 mmHg or diastolic blood pressure (DBP) >90 mmHg.

3. Single blood pressure (BP) >180/110 mmHg should be evaluated and treated immediately or within 1 week. (See **Tables 3-1 and 3-2.**[1])

Table 3-1. Classification of Blood Pressure

Category	Systolic (mmHg)	Diastolic (mmHg)
Optimal	<120	and <80
Prehypertension	120–139	or 80–89
Stage 1	140–159	or 90–99
Stage 2	≥160	or ≥100

Table 3-2. Cardiovascular Risk Factors

Major Risk Factors		Target Organ Damage	
Modifiable	•Age (men >55, women >65)	•Left ventricular hypertrophy (LVH)	•Angina / myocardial infarction (MI)
•Cigarette smoking	•Family history of CV disease (age: men <55 and women <65)		
•Dyslipidemia		•Coronary artery disease (CAD)	•Heart failure (HF)
•Obesity	•Diabetes mellitus	•Stroke or transient ischemic attack (TIA)	•Nephropathy
•Inactivity	•Microalbuminuria or glomerular filtration rate (GFR) <60 mL/min		•Retinopathy
		•Peripheral arterial disease	

Management

Lifestyle Modifications[1,3]

See Table 3-3.

Table 3-3. Lifestyle Modifications

Modification	Recommendation	Approx SBP (mmHg) Reduction
Weight loss	BMI 18.5–24.9	5–20 mmHg/10-kg weight loss
DASH plan	• Increase fruit, vegetables • Consume low-fat dairy with reduced saturated and total fat	8–14 mmHg
Sodium reduction	Limit to 2.4 g/day	2–8 mmHg

continued on next page

Table 3-3. Lifestyle Modifications (cont'd)

Modification	Recommendation	Approx SBP (mmHg) Reduction
Physical activity	Aerobic exercise or brisk walking at least 30 min/day 5 times weekly	4–9 mmHg
Moderation of alcohol intake	Limit to no more than 2 drinks/ day for men. Two drinks = • 1-oz or 30-mL ethanol • 24-oz beer • 10-oz wine • 3-oz 80 proof whiskey Limit to no more than 1 drink/ day for women and lighter persons	2–4 mmHg

Smoking cessation

General Treatment and Evaluation[1]

1. Assess patient understanding regarding therapy and barriers to adherence (physical, behavioral, education, understanding, attitude towards health). Using patient motivational interviewing techniques, assist the patient in setting goals that will address barriers to adherence. Develop an educational plan to address the issues assessed.

2. Lifestyle modifications are indicated for all patients with hypertension. They may be considered alone as treatment for patients with prehypertension. Review smoking cessation, basic nutrition, sodium reduction, cholesterol reduction, stress relief, and exercise. Consider referral to a nutritionist if indicated.

3. Identify the patient's goals and importance for taking medications.

4. Assess patient and first-degree history of relatives for cardiovascular disease or risk factors for cardiovascular disease (see Table 3-2).

5. Assess blood pressure and heart rate:

    a. Perform blood pressure measurement utilizing appropriate technique and blood pressure cuff size.

    b. Evaluate for presence of orthostatic hypotension.

6. Assess medication side effects, drug interactions, and food/lifestyle interactions.

7. Assess for medications or other substances that may exacerbate hypertension.

8. Assess and recognize signs of hypotension, hypertension, and end organ damage. Seek primary care provider consultation when necessary.

9. Monitor for improvement in symptoms if previously present (headaches, CP, SOB, angina).

10. Routine evaluation: Basic metabolic panel, renal function assessment, albumin/ creatinine ratio, fasting lipid panel, and, if appropriate, electrocardiogram (EKG).

11. Assess patient's physical characteristics and laboratory results to determine if pharmacokinetic properties of the antihypertensive medication require consideration.

12. Thiazide-type diuretic medications should be used as first-line agents for patients with uncomplicated hypertension. Thiazides may be used alone or in combination with other antihypertensive agents.

13. A majority of patients will require two or more antihypertensive agents to achieve BP goals.

14. Thiazide diuretics, ß-blockers, angiotensin-converting enzyme inhibitors (ACEI)/angiotensin II receptor blockers, and calcium-channel blockers are the only antihypertensive classes that have demonstrated, through randomized clinical trials, a reduction in mortality and morbidity from cardiovascular causes. The JNC-VII guidelines recommend thiazide diuretics and ACEI as first-line agents unless contraindicated, poorly tolerated, or special circumstances or compelling indications exist.

15. The evaluation of BP should occur within 2–4 weeks of starting therapy or 4–6 weeks for ACEI and reserpine. Assessment and monitoring for adverse effects should be performed routinely as problems usually present within 2–4 weeks of starting a drug or increasing the dose. After the patient is stable, BP monitoring can occur at intervals of 3–6 months and laboratory monitoring every 6–12 months unless additional monitoring is needed for concomitant conditions.[2]

Treatment Recommendations[1]

See Table 3-4.

Table 3-4. Guidelines for Treatment Initiation[1]

Classification	Lifestyle Modifications	Initial Drug Therapy	
		Without Compelling Indication	With Compelling Indication(s)
Normal	Yes	No drug therapy	No drug therapy
Prehypertension	Yes	No drug therapy	Drug(s) for the compelling indication(s)
Stage 1	Yes	Drug therapy: Thiazide for most. May consider ACEI, ARB, BB, CCB, or combination	Drug(s) for the compelling indication(s) Other antihypertensive drugs as needed
Stage 2*	Yes	Two drug combination for most. Drug therapy: Thiazide for most. May consider ACEI, ARB, BB, CCB, or combination	

continued on next page

* Stage 2 hypertension: Recognizing that patients with stage 2 hypertension will require two or more antihypertensive agents; consider initiating one antihypertensive agent initially to determine tolerability and then add the second agent or convert to a combination antihypertensive agent. If the patient requires two or more antihypertensive agents to maintain BP control, changing to the appropriate combination product may enhance medication adherence and reduce patient cost.

Compelling Indications for Drug Classes[1]

- CHF   ACEI, BB, Spironolactone, ARB, Thiazide
- Post MI   ACEI, BB, Spironolactone, ARB
- High CVD risk   Thiazide, ACEI, BB, CCB
- Diabetes without proteinuria   Thiazide, BB, ACEI, ARB, CCB
  and without heart disease
- Recurrent stroke prevention   Thiazide, ACEI

ACEI = angiotensin-converting enzyme inhibitor, BB = β-blocker, ARB = angiotensin II receptor blocker, CCB = long acting Ca-channel blocker

Other Compelling Indications for Drug Classes

- Diabetes with proteinuria   ARB, ACEI

  Meta-analysis suggests BP reduction (regardless of the agent utilized) provides renal and cardiovascular risk reduction.[4-9]

- Chronic renal disease   Thiazide, ACEI, ARB, BB[10,11]
- Elderly with LVH   BB, ARB,[12,13] possibly ACEI
- Elderly with LVH and ISH   ARB,[12,13] possibly ACEI
- Atrial fibrillation   BB, CCB (non-dihydropyridines)
- Angina   BB, CCB

Recommended Doses

- Refer to JNCVII guidelines[1]
- It is debatable if chlorthalidone is superior to hydrochlorothiazide. No comparative studies are available to determine if there is a difference in patient-oriented outcomes. The major thiazide studies have used chlorthalidone. Consider chlorthalidone or hydrochlorothiazide 12.5–25 mg daily.[14-16]

Causes for Resistant Hypertension[1]

- Improper BP measurement.
- Volume overload and pseudotolerance (excessive sodium intake, volume retention from kidney disease, inadequate diuretic therapy).
- Suboptimal pharmacotherapy (inadequate dose or inappropriate combinations, non-adherence).

- Drug-induced (NSAIDs, steroids, illicit drugs, sympathomimetics, oral contraceptives, herbal supplements, cyclosporine, tacrolimus, erythropoietin, licorice).
- Excessive alcohol use.
- Obesity.
- Identifiable co-morbidities (sleep apnea, chronic kidney disease, primary aldosteronism, reno-vascular disease, Cushing syndrome, pheochromocytoma, coarctation of the aorta, thyroid or parathyroid disease).

Possible Action for Resistant Hypertension

- Evaluate 24-hour ambulatory BP or home BP readings to detect the presence of white coat hypertension. If home BP or 24-hour ambulatory readings are elevated, treatment should be considered.
- Consider the addition of spironolactone 25–50 mg daily. Small studies suggest the addition of spironolactone in patients with resistant hypertension is effective. Monitor potassium and serum creatinine.
- Consider referral for evaluation of the mechanism of hypertension: volume versus vasoconstriction.[17]

Goals of Therapy

1. Reduce cardiovascular and renal morbidity and mortality.
2. Obtain target BP goals of < 140/90 mmHg or < 130/80 mmHg with diabetes or renal disease.

Clinical Pharmacy Goals

1. Identify patients with BP > 140/90 mmHg or > 130/80 mmHg if diabetes or renal disease.
2. Ensure patients with known hypertension obtain target BP goals of < 140/90 mmHg or < 130/80 mmHg with diabetes or renal disease.
3. Achieve target BP goals by utilizing thiazides as first-line agents unless contraindicated or compelling indications exist for another medication.
4. Guide and motivate the patient to be an active participant in his or her hypertension treatment and to actively participate in lifestyle modification.
5. Identify and address barriers to treatment adherence through demonstrating empathy and encouraging patient motivation.
6. Monitor for the presence of and reduce the incidence of medication side effects.
7. Identify and address potential causes of resistant hypertension.
8. Ensure patient understanding of hypertension, self-monitoring techniques, and appropriate follow-up.

Outcome Measures

1. Process measures: Patient has understanding of disease state and management principles; BP goals are achieved using the most cost-effective regimen.

2. Surrogate clinical markers: Patients with uncomplicated hypertension achieve BP control of <140/90 mmHg; patients with renal disease or diabetes achieve BP control of <130/80 mmHg.

3. Health outcome measures: Reduce the incidence of cardiovascular disease and associated morbidity and mortality.

Patient Information Resources

1. http://www.americanheart.org
2. http://www.nhlbi.nih.gov/guidelines/hypertension/

CASE STUDY

S: 56-yo black male presents for f/u of resistant hypertension. The primary care provider requests you review the medications and make recommendations. Upon reviewing the medication profile, you determine that he refills all medications on a monthly basis. He states that he is tolerating medications without side effects or difficulties. He is knowledgeable about the purpose, names, and doses of his medications. Uses a mediset box which, upon review, is filled appropriately. Reviewing the chart, you observe the patient's BP improved after each antihypertensive agent was added.

Hx: HTN, mild renal insufficiency, depression, MI 5 years ago.

Lifestyle: His diet is well balanced and consists of reasonable amounts of fruits and vegetables and low in sodium. Exercise is somewhat limited due to his hectic work/life schedule but walks 20 min 2–3 times weekly.

Review of systems: Pt denies SOB, CP, fatigue, vision changes, or weakness.

Medications:

HCTZ 25 mg q day

Lisinopril 40 mg q day

Nifedipine XL 90 mg q day

Metoprolol XL 200 mg q day

Lovastatin 40 mg q dinner

O: BP 158/94   HR 70

SCr 1.7 (stable for the past 3 years)

K 4.3   BUN 15

2002: LDL 186

2007: LDL 130

A/P:

Hypertension—uncontrolled on current regimen; goal BP <140/90

Dyslipidemia—uncontrolled on current regimen; goal LDL <100 mg/dL due to CAD

1. Add spironolactone 25 mg daily to treat resistant hypertension. *Current 4 antihypertensive regimen is maximized, and options are fairly limited. Reasonable options are adding spironolactone, clonidine, methyldopa, low-dose reserpine, or alpha-blocker. All are limited by specific side effects or difficult dosing adherence.*

2. Change lovastatin to simvastatin 40 mg daily for additional lipid lowering.

3. Encourage increase in walking regimen to 45 min 2–3 times weekly with goal of 45–60 min 4–5 times weekly.

4. Recheck SCr and K in 2 weeks (due to risk of developing hyperkalemia after starting spironolactone). Return to clinic for f/u in 4 weeks.

References

1. National High Blood Pressure Education Program Working Group. The seventh report of the Joint National Committee on prevention, dectection, evaluation and treatment of high blood pressure. *JAMA.* 2003; 289:2560–72. http://www.nhlbi.nih.gov/guidelines/hypertension/.

2. Saseen JJ, Carter BL. Hypertension. In: DiPiro JT, Talbert RL, Yee GC, et al, eds. *Pharmacotherapy: a pathophysiologic approach.* 6th ed. New York, NY: The McGraw-Hill Companies, Inc; 2005:185–217.

3. Smith SC, Allen J, Blair SN, et al. AHA/ACC guidelines for secondary prevention for patients with coronary and other atherosclerotic vascular disease: 2006 update. *Circulation.* 2006; 113:2363–72.

4. Cases JP, Chua W, Loukogeorgakis S, et al. Effect of inhibitors of the renin–angiotensin system and other antihypertensive drugs on renal outcomes: systematic review and meta-analysis. *Lancet.* 2005; 366:2026–33.

5. Strippoli G, Craig M, Deeks JJ, et al. Effects of angiotensin converting enzyme inhibitors and angiotensin II receptor antagonists on mortality and renal outcomes in diabetic nephropathy: systematic review. *BMJ.* 2004; 329:828.

6. Whelton PK, Barzilay J, Cushman W, et al. Clinical outcomes in antihypertensive treatment of type 2 diabetes, impaired fasting glucose concentration and normoglycemia. *Arch Intern Med.* 2005; 165:1401–9.

7. Berl T, Hunsicker LG, Lewis J, et al. Cardiovascular outcomes in the irbesartan diabetic nephropathy trial in patients with type 2 diabetes and overt nephropathy. *Arch Intern Med.* 2003; 138:542–9.

8. Lewis EJ, Hunsicker LG, Clarke WR, et al. Renoprotective effect of the angiotensin-receptor antagonist irbesartan in patients with nephropathy due to type 2 diabetes. *N Engl J Med.* 2001; 345:851–60.

9. Brenner BM, Cooper ME, deZeeuw D, et al. Effects of losartan on renal and cardiovascular outcomes in patients with type 2 diabetes and nephropathy. *N Engl J Med.* 2001; 345:861–9.

10. Rahman M, Pressel S, Davis B, et al. Renal outcomes in high-risk patients treated with an angiotension-converting enzyme inhibitor or a calcium channel blocker vs a diuretic. *Arch Intern Med.* 2005; 165:936–46.

11. Wright JT, Bakris G, Greene T, et al. Effect of blood pressure lowering and antihypertensive drug class on progression of hypertensive kidney disease: results from the AASK Trial. *JAMA.* 2002; 288:2421–31.

12. Dahlof B, Devereux RB, Kjeldsen SE, et al. Cardiovascular morbidity and mortality in the losartan intervention for endpoint reduction in hypertension study (LIFE): a randomized trial against atenolol. *Lancet.* 2002; 359:995–1003.

13. Kjeldsen SE, Dahlof B, Devereux RB, et al. Effects of losartan on cardiovascular morbidity and mortality in patients with isolated systolic hypertension and left ventricular hypertrophy: a losartan intervention for endpoint reduction (LIFE) substudy. *JAMA.* 2002; 288:1491–8.

14. ALLHAT Officers and Coordinators for the ALLHAT Collaborative Research Group. Major outcomes in high-risk hypertensive patients randomized to angiotensin-converting enzyme inhibitor or calcium channel blocker vs diuretic: the antihypertensive and lipid-lowering treatment to prevent heart attack trial (ALLHAT). *JAMA.* 2002; 288:2981–97.

15. Multiple Risk Factor Intervention Trial Research Group. Multiple risk factor intervention trial. Risk factor changes and mortality results. *JAMA.* 1982; 248:1465–77.

16. SHEP Cooperative Research Group. Prevention of stroke by antihypertensive drug treatment in older persons with isolated systolic hypertension. Final results of the systolic hypertension in the elderly program (SHEP). *JAMA.* 1991; 265:3255–64.

17. Taler S, Textor S, Augustine J. Resistant hypertension. Comparing hemodynamic management to specialist care. *Hypertension.* 2002; 39:982–8.

Diabetes Mellitus

Laura J. Hanson

Diabetes is a group of metabolic diseases characterized by hyperglycemia resulting from defects in insulin secretion, insulin action, or both. Diabetes affects approximately 20 million Americans; 90% of these patients have type 2 diabetes. The incidence of type 2 diabetes and its precursor, impaired glucose tolerance, continue to rise in the United States, paralleling the increase in overweight and obese Americans.[1] Pharmacists have the opportunity to participate in the care of diabetic patients in a variety of ways. Collaborative practice agreements allow pharmacists to be involved in the prevention and treatment of diabetes, its related co-morbid conditions, patient education, and facilitation of self-management skills in patients with diabetes.

Indications

Diabetes encompasses four classifications:

1. Type 1 diabetes (ß-cell destruction leading to absolute insulin deficiency).
2. Type 2 diabetes (progressive insulin secretory defect with background insulin resistance).
3. Specific types of diabetes due to other causes (genetic defects in ß-cell function, diseases of the pancreas, and drug- or chemical-induced diabetes).
4. Gestational diabetes mellitus (GDM).

While most patients referred to a pharmacist for diabetes management have been previously diagnosed, it is important to understand the criteria for diagnosis and risk factors necessitating screening as described in **Tables 4-1 and 4-2**.

Table 4-1. Criteria for Diagnosis of Diabetes

1) Symptoms of diabetes plus casual plasma glucose concentration ≥200 mg/dL. Casual is defined as any time of the day without regard to time since the last meal. The classic symptoms of diabetes include polyuria, polydipsia, and unexplained weight loss.

OR

2) Fasting plasma glucose ≥126 mg/dL. Fasting is defined as no caloric intake for at least 8 hours.

OR

3) 2-hour post load glucose ≥200 mg/dL during an oral glucose tolerance test. The test should be performed as described by WHO, using a glucose load containing the equivalent of 75 grams anhydrous glucose dissolved in water.

Table 4-2. Additional Risk Factors Considered for Screening Purposes

- Habitual physical inactivity
- Having a first-degree relative with diabetes
- Members of a high-risk ethnic population: African American, Latino, Native American, Asian American, Pacific Islander
- Delivering a baby weighing >9 lbs or having been diagnosed with GDM
- Hypertension (≥140/90 mmHg)
- HDL cholesterol <35 mg/dL and/or a triglyceride level >250 mg/dL
- Having polycystic ovarian syndrome (PCOS)
- Previous testing indicating impaired glucose tolerance (IGT) or impaired fasting glucose (IFG)
- Having other clinical conditions linked with insulin resistance (e.g., acanthosis nigricans)
- History of vascular disease

Management of Diabetes Mellitus

Treatment of diabetes must be individualized with equal emphasis on lifestyle modification and pharmacologic therapy. Normalization of blood sugar and prevention of microvascular and macrovascular complications are primary goals in all classes of diabetes. Large clinical trials have demonstrated that intensive therapy to normalize blood sugar levels results in decreased rates of retinopathy, nephropathy, and neuropathy.[2–4] Every 1% drop in hemoglobin A1c (HbA1c) is associated with improved clinical outcomes. However, these benefits must be weighed against the increased risk of severe hypoglycemia associated with intensive therapy.

Non-Pharmacologic Therapy

In addition to improving glycemic control, patients who change their lifestyle slow the progression of impaired glucose tolerance to overt diabetes.[5] Three major components to non-pharmacologic therapy in patients with diabetes include:

- Dietary modification with a low-calorie, low-fat, high carbohydrate diet
- Increased physical activity
- Weight reduction

Pharmacologic Therapy for Diabetes Mellitus

1. *Oral agents for glycemic control.* Oral agents are used in patients with type 2 diabetes, or other types of diabetes where functioning beta cells exist. There are currently four approaches to oral therapy for diabetes:

    a.   Increase insulin release with a sulfonylurea or meglitinide

    b.   Increase insulin responsiveness with a biguanide or thiazolidinedione

    c.   Decrease intestinal absorption of carbohydrate with an alpha-glucosidase inhibitor

    d.   Increase incretin hormones causing subsequent increase in insulin with sitagliptin

    These drugs are frequently combined to achieve therapeutic goals. Pharmacists should consider drug efficacy, side effects, and cost when selecting agents. Insulin therapy is frequently delayed secondary to concerns about hypoglycemia and patient willingness and/or ability to inject insulin.[6] However, avoiding insulin, the most potent of all hypoglycemic medications, may not be beneficial in the long term.

2. *Non-insulin injectable medications for glycemic control.* Glucose homeostasis is dependent on the interaction of multiple hormones: insulin and amylin, which are produced by pancreatic beta cells; glucagon, which is produced by pancreatic alpha cells; and gastrointestinal peptides, including glucagon-like peptide-1 (GLP-1) and gastric inhibitory peptide (GIP). Abnormal regulation of these substances may contribute to hyperglycemia.[7] Two new synthetic drugs, pramlintide (a synthetic analog of amylin) and exenatide (an incretin mimetic that exhibits similar actions to GLP-1), have recently been approved for use in the United States. These agents do not cause weight gain and do not cause hypoglycemia by themselves, but may increase the hypoglycemic effects of other agents when used in combination.

3. *Insulin therapy.* Insulin therapy is used to achieve tight glucose control to lower the frequency and severity of late-stage complications of diabetes, and to mimic the normal physiologic pattern of endogenous insulin secretion in healthy individuals. Insulin can be used in patients with all classes of

diabetes. All patients with type 1 diabetes require insulin at diagnosis, and many patients with type 2 diabetes will require insulin as their beta cell function declines over time. In type 2 diabetes, exogenously administered insulin may supplement relative endogenous insulin deficiency and help overcome insulin resistance.

Conventional insulin therapy. The term "conventional insulin therapy" has been used to describe more simple insulin regimens such as single daily injections, or two injections per day of regular and NPH insulin, mixed together in the same syringe and given in fixed amounts before breakfast and dinner. Conventional insulin therapy is unlikely to achieve target HbA1c levels in patients with type 1 diabetes, and may not provide adequate glycemic control for patients with type 2 diabetes.

Intensive insulin therapy. The term "intensive insulin therapy" is used to describe more complex regimens composed of long-acting basal insulin injection(s) and pre-meal doses of rapid-acting insulin given as three or more daily injections. While intensive regimens were initially used as therapy for type 1 diabetes, this strategy is now frequently used for patients with all types of diabetes. Current management strategies focus on replicating normal insulin secretion. Exogenous insulin is given to maintain a baseline insulin level between meals and at night, and rapidly rising insulin levels after meals (30–60 minutes), with a return to basal insulin concentrations within 2–3 hours.

Insulin initiation. Initial dose is largely dependent on provider experience and is adjusted soon after initiation based on the individual response. A reasonable starting point is based on the patient's weight (see **Table 4-3**). Differences in insulin efficacy, safety, and cost should be examined when selecting the initial insulin regimen. Basal insulin is usually given as 40–60% of the total daily dose, with the rest divided and given before meals. Obese patients with type 2 diabetes may require larger than expected insulin doses due to insulin resistance.[8]

a. Example insulin regimens for patients with type 1 diabetes

    i. Basal insulin

- Bedtime NPH with or without morning injection
- Glargine insulin

    ii. Prandial insulin

- Regular insulin may provide better blood sugar control for meals high in fat and protein due to longer duration of insulin action.
- Lispro and aspart may provide better control in high carbohydrate meals due to shorter duration of insulin action.

b. Example insulin regimens for patients with type 2 diabetes

Table 4-3. Weight-Based Insulin Dose

Usual Insulin Dose (units/kg actual body weight)

Type 1 Diabetes	0.2–0.6 units
Type 2 Diabetes, fasting BS 140–250 mg/dL	0.3–0.6 units
Type 2 Diabetes, fasting BS >250 mg/dL	0.5–1.5 units

i. Bedtime NPH has been shown to be an effective strategy for initiating insulin in patients already taking oral medications. This targets fasting glucose and subsequently lowers daytime blood sugar levels.

ii. Mixed regimen consisting of a pre-breakfast and pre-dinner dose of a long-acting insulin (e.g., NPH) and rapid-acting insulin (e.g., regular or lispro). Alternatively, it may be reasonable to consider commercially available premixed insulin (humulin 70/30) for convenience. If it is necessary to adjust the dose of fast-acting insulin before a meal, it is preferable to keep the fast-acting and intermediate-acting insulins as separate injections and adjust them independently.

iii. If patients are already taking an oral agent(s), may consider stopping therapy and converting patient to more intensive insulin regimen with basal and prandial insulin dosing.

Recommendations

All patients diagnosed with type 1 diabetes will require initiation of insulin therapy. If diet and exercise goals or the desired level of blood sugar control are not reached, patients with type 2 diabetes should be started on drug therapy. Either a sulfonylurea or metformin is a reasonable choice as a first-line agent, but the side effect profiles may favor metformin. The American Diabetes Association (ADA) and the European Association for the Study of Diabetes (EASD) issued a 2006 consensus statement for the management of type 2 diabetes.[9] Because of the difficulty in achieving and sustaining goal blood sugar control and significant weight loss, the consensus group concludes that metformin therapy should be initiated concurrent with lifestyle intervention at the time of diagnosis. Patients who are underweight, are losing weight, or are ketotic should always be started on insulin. Insulin can be considered an option for first-line therapy for all patients with type 2 diabetes.

If inadequate control is achieved with one oral medication, a second oral agent with a different mechanism of action or insulin should be started. Addition of insulin is recommended for patients whose HbA1c remains >8.5%, as it is unlikely that normoglycemia will be achieved by the addition of another oral agent.

Although three oral agents can be used, initiation and intensification of insulin therapy is preferred based on effectiveness and expense.[10] Pramlintide, exenatide, alpha-glucosidase inhibitors, and the meglitinides are not considered as second-line agents by the consensus panel due to limited clinical data, lower effectiveness in lowering glucose, and/or relatively greater expense.

Further adjustments of therapy, which should usually be made no less frequently than every 3 months, are based on the HbA1c result, aiming for levels as close to normal range as possible; with values >7%, the need for further adjustments in the diabetic regimen is suggested.

Self Blood Glucose Monitoring (SBGM)

Pharmacists frequently have the opportunity to educate patients on SBGM and glucometer use. All diabetic patients receiving drug therapy for blood sugar control should regularly monitor blood sugar; however, patients using insulin usually need to check blood sugar more often to prevent both hyperglycemia and hypoglycemia. The ADA recommends frequent monitoring, up to 4–6 times daily. SBGM is extremely valuable in patients using insulin because they experience daily variability in blood glucose levels. Many factors including exercise, stress, illness, hormonal changes, and travel can affect blood sugar levels. Frequent SBGM is necessary to adjust insulin therapy and achieve goal glycemic control.

Diabetic Self-Management Education (DSME)

Standards for diabetes self-management education (DSME) have been developed by the American Diabetes Association. DSME has been shown to be most effective when delivered by a multidisciplinary team with a comprehensive plan of care.

Appropriately trained pharmacists can help patients with diabetes understand their disease state, and more effectively participate in their own care. The individual needs of patients should be considered to help determine what areas of diabetes education are appropriate. The recommendations for DSME are reviewed and revised regularly. The following written curriculum has been recommended by the ADA.[11]

- Describing the diabetes disease process and treatment options
- Incorporating appropriate nutritional management
- Incorporating physical activity into lifestyle
- Utilizing medications for therapeutic effectiveness
- Monitoring blood glucose and urine ketones (when appropriate) as well as using the results to improve control
- Preventing, detecting, and treating acute complications
- Preventing (through risk-reduction behavior), detecting, and treating chronic complications

- Goal setting to promote health and problem solving for daily living
- Integrating psychosocial adjustment to daily life
- Promoting preconception care, management during pregnancy, and gestational diabetes management (if applicable)

Management of Comorbid Conditions

Hypertension

Early treatment of high blood pressure is important in the prevention of cardiovascular disease and to minimize the rate of progression of diabetic nephropathy and retinopathy.[12] Lifestyle modification is the preferred initial therapy in the absence of renal disease or high risk of cardiovascular disease. This lifestyle modification includes weight reduction, increased exercise, sodium restriction, smoking cessation, and limiting alcohol consumption.

For patients with diabetes, the choice of antihypertensive agent(s) is based upon prevention of adverse cardiovascular events. The agents also serve to slow the progression of existing renal disease.

- ALLHAT found that high-risk patients, including those with diabetes, have a better cardiovascular outcome with a thiazide diuretic than with an angiotensin-converting enzyme inhibitor (ACEI).[13]
- ACEIs and angiotensin receptor blockers (ARBs) protect against the development of progressive nephropathy due to type 1 and 2 diabetes.[14,15] However, the choice of one of these agents for initial monotherapy does not have great clinical relevance, because combination therapy with a diuretic and an ACEI or ARB will be required in almost all patients with hypertension and diabetes to attain goal blood pressure values.
- Based upon ALLHAT, individuals with diabetes and hypertension are started on a low-dose thiazide diuretic unless there is an indication for another antihypertensive agent. If low-dose thiazide monotherapy is inadequate to attain goal blood pressure, an ACEI or ARB should be added. Combination therapy is required for the majority of patients.[16] If an ACEI is not tolerated, an ARB should be substituted.

Hyperlipidemia

The National Cholesterol Education Program report from the United States and guidelines from Europe consider type 2 diabetes to be a coronary heart disease (CHD) equivalent, elevating it to the highest risk category.[17] This classification is based in part upon the observation that patients with type 2 diabetes without a prior myocardial infarction (MI) are at the same risk for MI and coronary mortality as patients without diabetes who had a prior myocardial infarction.[18]

At any cholesterol level, patients with diabetes have more coronary disease than nondiabetic patients. This increase in risk may be due to qualitative differences in the lipoprotein fractions or to the presence of other proatherosclerotic metabolic changes. The association of elevated LDL cholesterol with cardiovascular risk in many epidemiologic studies has been reinforced by randomized clinical trials showing that statin therapy improves outcomes in diabetics, including those without clinical evidence of CHD.[19]

Antiplatelet Therapy

- Aspirin therapy (75–162 mg/day) is recommended as secondary prevention in all patients with diabetes and a history of cardiovascular disease (CVD).[20]

- Aspirin therapy (75–162 mg/day) is recommended as primary prevention in patients with type 1 or type 2 diabetes and increased CVD risk (individuals >40 years old, family history of CVD, hypertension, smoking, dyslipidemia, albuminuria).

- May consider aspirin therapy in patients between 30 and 40 years old with CVD risk factors.

- Aspirin therapy should not be used in patients under the age of 21 due to the increased risk of Reye's syndrome.

- Combination therapy with other antiplatelet agents in addition to aspirin should be used in patients with severe and/or progressive CVD.

- Other antiplatelet agents may be used alternatively in patients who cannot take aspirin due to allergy, recent GI bleed, etc.

Smoking Cessation

A recent survey completed in the United States found that the prevalence of cigarette smoking was higher among diabetic patients than nondiabetic subjects, even after adjusting for age, sex, race, and educational level.[21] Over 25% of patients newly diagnosed with diabetes were smokers. A meta-analysis of many of the cardiovascular risk reduction trials showed that cessation of smoking had a much greater benefit on survival than most other interventions.[22] These findings suggest that smoking cessation is one of the most important aspects of therapy in patients with diabetes.

Vaccination

Patients with diabetes mellitus should receive influenza vaccination yearly and a pneumococcal vaccination, repeating the pneumococcal vaccine once after age 65 years if the initial vaccination was prior to age 65. Tetanus and diphtheria vaccinations should also be updated.[20]

Goals of Therapy

1. Near normalization of blood glucose appropriate to individual patient circumstances as measured by a standardized HbA1c.

    a. HbA1c measured every 3 months (may be monitored less frequently in patients meeting treatment goals).

    b. HbA1c goal in general should be ≤7%. The HbA1c goal for the individual patient is as close to normal (<6%) as possible without significant hypoglycemia. A higher target may be chosen for patients at severe risk of hypoglycemia or with minimal benefit from tight control (elderly patients, young children, etc).

2. Pre-prandial capillary plasma glucose 90–130 mg/dL

3. Blood pressure ≤130/80 mmHg (see Chapter 3 for further discussion of hypertension management)

4. Lipid management

    a. LDL <100 mg/dL, triglycerides <150 mg/dL, and HDL >50 mg/dL.

    b. In people with diabetes over the age of 40 with a total cholesterol ≥135 mg/dL, recommending statin therapy to achieve an LDL reduction of approximately 30%, regardless of baseline LDL levels, may be appropriate.[23]

    c. See Chapter 2 for further discussion of dyslipidemia management.

5. Cardiovascular risk reduction

    a. Antiplatelet therapy in appropriate individuals

    b. Weight reduction

    c. Smoking cessation (see Chapter 8 for discussion of smoking cessation)

6. Prevention of diabetic complications

    a. Retinopathy, nephropathy, neuropathy, and cardiovascular disease

    See **Table 4-4**.

Clinical Pharmacy Goals

1. Identify patients not meeting pharmacologic treatment goals (HbA1C, high blood pressure, hyperlipidemia, etc.) and optimize treatment using cost-effective therapy to achieve goals.

2. Identify appropriate patients not on antiplatelet therapy and initiate most appropriate agent or agents.

3. Identify patients using tobacco and recommend/facilitate smoking cessation.

4. Facilitate education of self-care, self-blood sugar monitoring, and understanding of diabetes and potential complications.

Table 4-4. Monitoring and Evaluation

Data Elements	Frequency
Age at diagnosis	Once
Health habits (alcohol, exercise, smoking)	Yearly
Obesity (screening)	Every 3 years
Glycosylated hemoglobin (HbA1c)	Every 3 months; may consider less frequent monitoring in patients meeting treatment goals
Ophthalmology visit (dilated eye exam)	Yearly; may consider less frequent exams in low-risk patients on the advice of an eye care professional
Urine protein, albumin screening	Yearly
Foot exam, PAD screening	Yearly
Blood pressure (screening)	At each routine visit for diabetes
Fasting lipid profile	Yearly, or every 2 years in patients meeting goals
Influenza vaccine	Yearly
Pneumococcal vaccine	Once or repeated according to guidelines
CHD screening, risk assessment	Yearly
Tobacco use assessment	At each routine visit

5. Ensure all patients are able to demonstrate proper glucometer technique.

6. Identify and follow up patients with high emergency department or urgent care use for diabetes-related visits.

Outcome Measures

1. Surrogate clinical markers: Achieve pharmacologic treatment goals:
   a. HbA1c <7%
   b. Blood pressure <130/80
   c. LDL <100 mg/dL

2. Health outcome measures: Reduction in number of visits to the emergency department and/ or urgent care clinic for diabetes-related problems; reduction in hospitalizations for diabetes complications; reduction in cardiovascular events.

Patient Information Resources

1. http://www.diabetes.org

CASE STUDY

S: 45-year-old African American male referred to pharmacist for repeat fingerstick and possible initiation of pharmacologic therapy for suspected diabetes. PMH includes HTN and obesity. Pt had an appointment with his provider last week, and was noted to have an elevated fasting blood sugar (BS) of 128 mg/dL. He reports being told that he was "pre-diabetic" in the past, but did not follow up because he did not want to "give himself shots." He has been taking HCTZ 25 mg daily for ~ 1 year and reports taking this regularly. He checks his BP occasionally, and thinks that it usually runs in the 130s/80s and is "good." He denies chest pain, dyspnea, edema, headaches, and dizziness. He describes a diet with frequent fast food meals, and reports a 15 lb weight gain over the last year. He does not pay attention to caloric intake, dietary fats, or salt in his diet. He reports a sedentary lifestyle, but plans to start exercising in the spring. He wonders today if his BP medication could be making him urinate more frequently. He forgot to mention this to his physician last week, but remembers his HCTZ causing this when he first started taking it. He complains of increased fatigue, having to get up at night 3–4 times to urinate, and "itchy skin."

Family History: + mother with diabetes, + father with hypertension and CAD, both deceased. No siblings.

Social History: –tobacco use, 1–2 beers daily with dinner, no history of illegal drug use

Allergies: NKDA

Current medications:

   HCTZ 25 mg daily

   Multiple vitamin daily

   OTC athlete's foot product

O:

VS: BP 139/89; HR 80/min and reg; Wt 120 kg, RR 16/min, Temp 98

Labs checked this AM:

Chemistry panel: Glu 280, SCr 1.4, other values wnl

LFTs wnl

Fasting lipids: LDL 190, HDL 30, TG 220

HbA1c: 8%

A:

1. Diabetes. Pt with newly diagnosed type 2 diabetes mellitus, appropriate to start drug therapy at this time. *Signs and symptoms of hyperglycemia along with elevated casual BS measured today are sufficient for diagnosis. Also recent high BS value measured in clinic. Although not diagnostic, elevated HbA1c discovered. Multiple risk factors present.*

2. Hypertension: Not at goal blood pressure (<130/80 mmHg) on current regimen. High sodium diet, recent weight gain, and physical inactivity may be contributory.

3. Hyperlipidemia: Elevated cholesterol, no history of CAD, new diagnosis of diabetes mellitus. Goal LDL <100 mg/dL. Not likely to be achieved by lifestyle modification alone. Cholesterol panel may improve with better blood sugar control, but will require drug therapy to meet LDL goal.

P:

1. Diabetes

    a. Discussed diabetes mellitus, risk factors for disease, possible diabetic complications, and importance of normalizing BS. Plan to start low-dose metformin 500 mg BID today, and titrate as necessary for blood sugar control and goal HbA1c <7%. *Pt is overweight and may benefit from expected weight stabilization or weight loss with metformin treatment. Pt has somewhat elevated serum creatinine, but has adequate creatinine clearance for safe metformin use. Metformin is initial choice for drug therapy based on 2006 consensus recommendations.*[9]

    b. Demonstrated proper glucometer technique at this visit. Pt able to repeat instructions and perform own self BS monitoring today. Agrees to twice daily monitoring, fasting, and before bedtime until next visit.

    c. Cardiovascular risk reduction: Add ASA 81 mg daily; recommend increased physical activity and dietary changes to facilitate weight loss.

    d. Patient education: Will require more extensive diabetes education at future f/u visits. Pt will need additional information about diabetes complications and risk reduction, following a diabetic diet, sick day management, foot care, and oral hygiene. Plan to f/u with patient regularly. Will refer to nutrition and available diabetes classes for additional education.

e. Laboratory: Pt to have Alb/Cr ratio checked before next f/u visit.

f. Refer to podiatry and ophthalmology for annual examination.

g. Vaccinations: Recommend annual influenza vaccination and pneumococcal vaccination.

2. Hypertension: Add lisinopril 5 mg daily, repeat chemistry panel in 2 weeks. *Patient is already taking a thiazide diuretic with inadequate control; available evidence suggests that addition of an ACEI may prevent or delay progression of diabetic nephropathy. Lisinopril is available as a generic and is a cost-effective addition.*

3. Hyperlipidemia: Add lovastatin 40 mg daily and dietary modification. Repeat fasting lipid panel in 6–8 weeks.

4. Follow-up visit scheduled in 1 week with pharmacist for diabetes management and hypertension f/u. Pt verbalized understanding plan for medication changes and monitoring. No further questions at this time.

References

1. Killilea T. Long-term consequences of type 2 diabetes mellitus: economic impact on society and managed care. *Am J Manag Care.* 2002; 8:S441–9.

2. The Diabetes Control and Complications Trial Research Group. The effect of intensive treatment of diabetes on the development and progression of long-term complications in insulin-dependent diabetes mellitus. *N Engl J Med.* 1993; 329:977.

3. UK Prospective Diabetes Study (UKPDS) Group. Intensive blood-glucose control with sulfonylureas or insulin compared with conventional treatment and risk of complications in patients with type 2 diabetes (UKPDS 33). *Lancet.* 1998; 352:837.

4. Ohkubo Y, Kishikawa H, Araki E, et al. Intensive insulin therapy prevents the progression of diabetic microvascular complications in Japanese patients with non-insulin-dependent diabetes mellitus: A randomized prospective 6-year study. *Diabetes Res Clin Pract.* 1995; 28:103.

5. Knowler WC, Barrett-Connor E, Fowler SE, et al. Reduction in the incidence of type 2 diabetes with lifestyle intervention or metformin. *N Engl J Med.* 2002; 346:393.

6. Hirsch IB, Bergenstal RM, Parkin CG, et al. A real-world approach to insulin therapy in primary care practice. *Clin Diabetes.* 2005; 23:78–86.

7. Riddle MC, Drucker DJ. Emerging therapies mimicking the effects of amylin and glucagon-like peptide 1. *Diabetes Care.* 2006; 29:435–8.

8. Hirsch IB, Vega CP. Optimal initiation of insulin in type 2 diabetes. *Med Gen Med.* 2005; 7(4):49.

9. Nathan DM, Buse JB, Davidson MB, et al. Management of hyperglycemia in type 2 diabetes: a consensus algorithm for the initiation and adjustment of therapy: a consensus statement from the American Diabetes Association and the European Association for the Study of Diabetes. *Diabetes Care.* 2006; 29:1963.

10. Sheehan MT. Current therapeutic options in type 2 diabetes mellitus: a practical approach. *Clin Med Res.* 2003; 1:189–200.

11. National Standards for Diabetes Self-Management Education. *Diabetes Care.* 2006; 29:S78–85.

12. Adler AI, Stratton IM, Neil HA, et al. Association of systolic blood pressure with macrovascular and microvascular complications of type 2 diabetes (UKPDS 36): prospective observational study. *BMJ.* 2000; 321:412.

13. Major outcomes in high-risk hypertensive patients randomized to angiotensin-converting enzyme inhibitor or calcium channel blocker vs diuretic: the Antihypertensive and Lipid-Lowering Treatment to Prevent Heart Attack Trial (ALLHAT). *JAMA.* 2002; 288:2981.

14. Lindholm LH, Ibsen H, Dahlof B, et al. Cardiovascular morbidity and mortality in patients with diabetes in the Losartan Intervention for Endpoint reduction in hypertension study (LIFE): a randomized trial against atenolol. *Lancet.* 2002; 359:1004.

15. The Microalbuminuria Captopril Study Group. Captopril reduces the risk of nephropathy in IDDM patients with microalbuminuria. *Diabetologia.* 1996; 39:587.

16. Chobanian AV, Bakris GL, Black HR, et al. The Seventh Report of the Joint National Committee on Prevention, Detection, Evaluation, and Treatment of High Blood Pressure: The JNC 7 Report. *JAMA.* 2003; 289:2560.

17. Third Report of the National Cholesterol Education Program (NCEP) Expert Panel on Detection, Evaluation, and Treatment of High Blood Cholesterol in Adults (Adult Treatment Panel III) final report. *Circulation.* 2002; 106:3143.

18. Haffner SM, Lehto S, Ronnemaa T, et al. Mortality from coronary heart disease in subjects with type 2 diabetes and in nondiabetic subjects with and without prior myocardial infarction. *N Engl J Med.* 1998; 339:229.

19. Yudkin JS. How can we best prolong life? Benefits of coronary risk factor reduction in non-diabetic and diabetic subjects. *BMJ.* 1993; 306:1313.

20. American Diabetes Association: Standards of Medical Care in Diabetes—2006. *Diabetes Care.* 2006; (29 Suppl):S1–S85.

21. Ford ES, Malarcher AM, Herman WH, et al. Diabetes mellitus and cigarette smoking: findings from the 1989 National Health Interview Survey. *Diabetes Care.* 1994; 17:688.

22. Yudkin JS. How can we best prolong life? Benefits of coronary risk factor reduction in non-diabetic and diabetic subjects. *BMJ.* 1993; 306:1313.

23. Heart Protection Study Collaborative Group. MRC/BHF Heart Protection Study of cholesterol lowering with simvastatin in 20,536 high-risk individuals: a randomized placebo-controlled trial. *Lancet.* 2002; 360:7–22.

Thromboembolic Disorders

Greta Sweney

Arterial and venous thrombosis are major causes of mortality. Each year about 700,000 people experience a new or recurrent stroke; of these, 87% are ischemic strokes.[1] In addition, up to 2 million venous thromboembolic events (VTEs), including deep vein thrombosis (DVT) and pulmonary embolism (PE), occur annually leading to significant morbidity and mortality.[2] Pharmacists play an important role in care for patients with thromboembolic disorders. Studies have shown that an anticoagulation clinic can be cost effective and significantly decrease bleeding and thromboembolic events.[3]

Indications

Patients with documented thromboembolic disorders requiring anticoagulation therapy will be referred by their primary providers to the clinical pharmacist for management and education. Refer to **Table 5-1** for indications for anticoagulation, target International Normalized Ratio (INR), and recommended duration of therapy.

Management

1. Verify the indication and treatment option are appropriate for anticoagulation therapy.
2. Perform medical history, limited physical exam, and medication review to determine risks of bleeding and thromboembolic events.
3. Determine antithrombotic agent (warfarin, heparin, low molecular weight heparin, or a combination) and initiate therapy.

Table 5-1. Optimal Therapeutic Range and Duration of Anticoagulation

INDICATION	TARGET INR (RANGE)	DURATION	COMMENT
ATRIAL FIBRILLATION (AF)/ATRIAL FLUTTER			
Age < 65 with no risk factors	*none*	chronic	use aspirin 325mg qd alone
Age 65–75 with no risk factors	2.5 (2.0 – 3.0)	chronic	or aspirin 325mg qd
age > 75 OR any risk factor	2.5 (2.0 – 3.0)	chronic	
[hx TIA/stroke/TE; HTN; poor LV fxn; mitral valve dz; valve replacement]			
pre cardioversion (Afib or flutter > 48 hours)	2.5 (2.0 – 3.0)	3 weeks	
post cardioversion (in NSR)	2.5 (2.0 – 3.0)	4 weeks	
CARDIOEMBOLIC STROKE			
with risk factors for stroke	2.5 (2.0 – 3.0)	chronic	
[AF, CHF, LV dysfxn; mural thrombus, hx TIA/stroke/TE]			
following embolic event despite antico agulation	2.5 (2.0 – 3.0)	chronic	add antiplatelet therapy
LEFT VENTRICULAR DYSFUNCTION (LV DSYFXN)			
ejection fraction < 30%	2.5 (2.0 – 3.0)	chronic	
transient, following myocardial infarction	2.5 (2.0 – 3.0)	3 months	and aspirin 81mg qd
following embolic event despite anticoagulation	2.5 (2.0 – 3.0)	chronic	add antiplatelet therapy
MYOCARDIAL INFARCTION (MI)			
following anterior MI	2.5 (2.0 – 3.0)	3 months	and aspirin 81mg qd
following inferior MI with transient risk(s)	2.5 (2.0 – 3.0)	3 months	and aspirin 81mg qd
[AF; CHF, LV dysfxn, mural thrombus, hx TE]			
following initial tx with persistent risks	2.5 (2.0 – 3.0)	chronic	and aspirin 81mg qd
THROMBOEMBOLISM (DVT, PE)	**(preceded by UFH/LMWH for min 5 days and until INR > 2)**		
	(for DVT, add elastic compression stockings with 30 – 40mmHg at ankle for 2 years)		
treatment/prevention of recurrence (including calf vein and upper extremity DVT)			
transient risk factors	2.5 (2.0 – 3.0)	3 months	
idiopathic/first episode	2.5 (2.0 – 3.0)	6 – 12 months	consider chronic therapy
recurrent VTE	2.5 (2.0 – 3.0)	chronic	
with malignancy	2.5 (2.0 – 3.0)	chronic	preceded by LMWH x 3 – 6 mo
hypercoagulable state	2.5 (2.0 – 3.0)	6 – 12 months	consider chronic therapy
two or more thrombophilic conditions	2.5 (2.0 – 3.0)	12 months	consider chronic therapy
antiphospholipid antibody (APA) syndrome	2.5 (2.0 – 3.0)	12 months	consider chronic therapy
~ with recurrent VTE or other risk factors	3.0 (2.5 – 3.5)	12 months	consider chronic therapy
chronic thromboembolic pulmonary hypertension	2.5 (2.0 – 3.0)	chronic	
cerebral venous sinus thrombosis	2.5 (2.0 – 3.0)	3 – 6 months	
VALVULAR DISEASE			
aortic valve disease			
with mobile atheroma or aortic plaque > 4mm	2.5 (2.0 – 3.0)	chronic	
mitral valve prolapse, regurgitation, or annular calcification			
with AF or hx systemic embolization	2.5 (2.0 – 3.0)	chronic	
with recurrent TIA despite ASA therapy	2.5 (2.0 – 3.0)	chronic	
rheumatic mitral valve disease:			
with AF, hx systemic embolization, or LA > 5.5cm	2.5 (2.0 – 3.0)	chronic	
s/p embolic event despite anticoagulatio n	2.5 (2.0 – 3.0)	chronic	add aspirin 81mg qd
VALVE REPLACEMENT – BIOPROSTHETIC			
aortic	2.5 (2.0 – 3.0)	3 months	followed by aspirin (or aspirin alone)
mitral	2.5 (2.0 – 3.0)	3 months	followed by aspirin 81mg qd
aortic or mitral			
with LA thrombus	2.5 [2.0 – 3.0]	> 3 months	followed by aspirin 81mg qd
with prior history systemic embolism	2.5 [2.0 – 3.0]	3 – 12 months	followed by aspirin 81mg qd
with atrial fibrillation	2.5 [2.0 – 3.0]	chronic	
following systemic embolism	2.5 [2.0 – 3.0]	chronic	add aspirin 81mg qd
VALVE REPLACEMENT – MECHANICAL			
aortic bileaflet St Jude	2.5 (2.0 – 3.0)	chronic	
bileaflet Carbomedics/tilting disk Medronic Hall			
~in NSR, with nl EF, and nl LA size	2.5 (2.0 – 3.0)	chronic	
~all others	3.0 (2.5 – 3.5)	chronic	
tilting disk (all other brands)	3.0 (2.5 – 3.5)	chronic	
ball and cage/caged disk	3.0 (2.5 – 3.5)	chronic	with aspirin 81mg qd
mitral bileaflet or tilting disk	3.0 (2.5 – 3.5)	chronic	
ball and cage/caged disk	3.0 (2.5 – 3.5)	chronic	with aspirin 81mg qd
with additional risk factors or following TE event	3.0 (2.5 – 3.5)	chronic	add aspirin 81mg qd

4. Provide anticoagulation education, teaching, and consultation to patients and medical staff.

5. Based on the antithrombotic agent initiated, follow up and monitor appropriate laboratory tests at indicated time intervals.

6. Adjust dose as necessary to maintain therapeutic anticoagulation.

7. Manage over-anticoagulation and under-anticoagulation as needed.

8. Evaluate for discontinuation of anticoagulation therapy when appropriate.

Heparin

Prior to the introduction of low molecular weight heparins (LMWHs), unfractionated heparin (UFH) was the standard for initial treatment of all thromboembolic disorders. Treatment doses of heparin are typically weight based and vary with the indication for use. Careful monitoring is essential, as it has a narrow therapeutic window and an unpredictable dose response.[4] The activated partial thromboplastin time (aPTT) should be monitored, heparin adjusted, and maintained in the therapeutic range per established protocol. Due to the wide variation in testing reagents and instruments, the therapeutic range and resulting dose adjustments should be modified for each institution.

Complications from UFH include:

- Bleeding
- Osteoporosis
- Heparin-induced thrombocytopenia (HIT)

The anticoagulant effects of heparin can be reversed with protamine. Heparin-induced thrombocytopenia should be managed with direct thrombin inhibitors. For detailed information, see the Seventh American College of Chest Physicians (ACCP) Conference on Antithrombotic and Thrombolytic Therapy: Evidence-Based Guidelines.[4]

Low Molecular Weight Heparin (LMWH)

LMWHs are isolated shorter heparin molecules with a lower molecular weight compared to UFH. Each LMWH is derived by a different chemical method and has a different molecular weight, yet all have good bioavailability and superior pharmacokinetic properties. Currently, three LMWH products are available in the United States: enoxaparin, dalteparin, and tinzaparin. These products are administered in fixed doses for prophylaxis and total body weight (TBW) adjusted doses for treatment of a thromboembolic event. Laboratory monitoring is generally not required for LMWH, except in special populations such as renal patients, obese patients, or pregnant patients.

1. General dosing guidelines
   a. Initial treatment of acute thrombosis
      i. Enoxaparin 1 mg/kg subcutaneously q 12 h for minimum course of 5 days and until INR is in therapeutic range for 2 consecutive days. Enoxaparin 1.5 mg/kg q 24 h may also be used in patients who are not obese (BMI >27) and who do not have malignancy.[5]
      ii. Tinzaparin 175 anti-Xa International Units (IU)/kg subcutaneously daily for a minimum course of 6 days and until INR is in therapeutic range for 2 consecutive days.[6]
      iii. Dalteparin 200 IU/kg subcutaneously q 24 h for a minimum of 5 days

and until INR is in therapeutic range for 2 consecutive days. (This dose is used internationally and not FDA approved for this indication.)

b. Initial anticoagulation in patients with atrial fibrillation, heart valve replacement, LV thrombus, or other cardiovascular indications for anticoagulation

    i. Enoxaparin 1 mg/kg subcutaneously q 12 h[5]

    ii. Dalteparin 120 IU/kg q 12 h (FDA approved only for acute myocardial infarction, ST-segment elevations, and unstable angina)[7]

c. Dosing in the obese patient

Most LMWH clinical trials have excluded patients above 150 kilograms. The current recommendation is to dose LMWH based on TBW and monitor anti-factor Xa levels for patients greater than 150 kg.

d. Dosing for renal insufficiency

A linear relationship between anti-factor Xa plasma clearance and creatinine clearance (CrCl) at steady state has been observed; thus, patients with decreased CrCl also have decreased LMWH clearance.[4] If patients have a moderate decrease in CrCl (<60 mL/min), use LMWH with caution and monitor anti-factor Xa levels. In patients with a CrCl <30 mL/min, LMWH is not recommended except for enoxaparin, which has dosing recommendations available for patients with renal impairment.

e. Dosing in pregnancy

Warfarin is teratogenic and should be avoided during pregnancy. Use adjusted dose UFH or LMWH to prevent or treat thromboembolic events before or during pregnancy. Dosing of LMWH is based on TBW at appropriate doses for prevention or treatment. Monitoring anti-factor Xa levels may be necessary.

f. Short-term monitoring guidelines for all LMWH

    i. Platelet count: every 2–3 days during first 14 days of therapy.

    ii. Peak anti-factor Xa activity if appropriate:

        • 3–4 hours after dose in patients with:

           - Renal impairment (CrCl <60 mL/min)

           - Obesity (wt >150 kg)

           - Unexpected hemorrhage

        • Check after third dose and again if adjustment required

        • Goal:

           - 0.5–1.0 units/mL for bid dosing

           - 1.0–2.0 units/mL for daily dosing

    iii. Trough anti-factor Xa monitoring may be indicated to evaluate accumulation.

        • Measure at end of dosing interval

- Check before fourth dose and again if adjustment required
- Goal: <0.5 units/mL

g. Long-term monitoring guidelines for all LMWH

In some instances, such as pregnancy or a thromboembolic event in patients with cancer, LMWH may be used for months. It is appropriate to monitor the following and adjust dose as necessary:

i. Peak anti-factor Xa activity: once monthly

ii. Serum creatinine (SCr): once monthly

iii. Creatinine clearance (CrCl): calculate monthly

iv. Patient weight: check monthly

v. Platelets: once monthly

vi. Hematocrit (Hct): once monthly

vii. Bone mineral density during prolonged therapy

Warfarin

The vitamin K antagonists (VKAs) have been the standard of oral anticoagulation for more than 50 years.[4] Warfarin is the VKA available in the United States. The effectiveness of warfarin is strongly established in well designed clinical trials for most of the indications listed in Table 5-1.[4] Warfarin may be challenging to manage due to:

- A narrow therapeutic window
- Considerable variability in dose response among patients
- Interactions with drugs and diet
- Laboratory controls that can be difficult to standardize
- Dosing problems that occur as a result of patient non-adherence and miscommunication between patient and anticoagulation provider[4]

The flexible initiation method and the average daily dosing method are the two most common approaches used to initiate warfarin therapy. Using nomograms (see **Tables 5-2** and **5-3**) as a guide, the goal is to avoid over-anticoagulation and under-anticoagulation. Over-anticoagulation increases the risk of hemorrhage, while under-anticoagulation may prolong a hospital stay or the need for parenteral anticoagulants or it may precipitate a thrombotic event. Rapid anticoagulation happens with the reduction of three of the vitamin K dependent factors, approximately 6–24 hours after initiating therapy, but the reduction of prothrombin (factor II) has a longer half life (approximately 60–72 hours), so it takes about 4 days to see the full anticoagulation effect. Due to this delay in the anticoagulation effect, when rapid anticoagulation effect is needed, it is recommended to overlap heparin or LMWH with warfarin for at least 4 days and until the INR is within the therapeutic range for 2 days.[4,8]

Table 5-2. Flexible Initiation Method

Day	INR	5-mg Initiation DOSE	10-mg Initiation DOSE
1	–	5 mg	10 mg
2	<1.5	5 mg	7.5–10 mg
	1.5–1.9	2.5 mg	2.5 mg
	2.0–2.5	1.0–2.5 mg	1.0–2.5 mg
	>2.5	0	0
3	<1.5	5–10 mg	5–10 mg
	1.5–1.9	2.5–5 mg	2.5–5 mg
	2.0–2.5	0–2.5 mg	0–2.5 mg
	2.5–3.0	0–2.5 mg	0–2.5 mg
	>3.0	0	0
4	<1.5	10 mg	10 mg
	1.5–1.9	5–7.5 mg	5–7.5 mg
	2.0–3.0	0–5 mg	0–5 mg
	>3.0	0	0
5	<1.5	10 mg	10 mg
	1.5–1.9	7.5–10 mg	7.5–10 mg
	2.0–3.0	0–5 mg	0–5 mg
	>3.0	0	0
6	<1.5	7.5–12.5 mg	7.5–12.5 mg
	1.5–1.9	5–10 mg	5–10 mg
	2.0–3.0	0–7.5 mg	0–7.5 mg
	>3.0	0	0

Table 5-3. Average Daily Dosing Method

	Non-Sensitive Patients	Sensitive Patients*
Initial Dose	5 mg q day	2.5 mg q day
First INR	3 days	3 days
<1.5	7.5 mg q day	5 mg q day
1.5–1.9	5 mg q day	2.5 mg q day
2–3	2.5 mg q day	1.25 mg q day
3.1–4	1.25 mg q day	0.5 mg q day
>4	Hold	Hold
Next INR	2–3 days	2–3 days

* Factors that influence sensitivity to warfarin: age >75, clinical congestive heart failure, diarrhea, drug interactions that decrease warfarin metabolism, elevated baseline INR, fever, hyperthyroidism, malignancy, malnutrition, or NPO >3 days.

Flexible Initiation Method

The nomogram in Table 5-2 is useful in hospitalized patients in which an INR can be checked each day. Two randomized clinical trials have suggested that 5-mg initiation achieves therapeutic anticoagulation as rapidly as 10-mg initiation but with a lower frequency of supratherapeutic INRs.[9,10] The 10-mg initiation nomogram should only be used in relatively young and healthy patients who are likely to be insensitive to warfarin, or in patients taking concurrent medications known to induce warfarin metabolism.

Average Daily Dosing Method

The nomogram in Table 5-3 illustrates the average daily dosing method of warfarin initiation, which is particularly useful for ambulatory patients and is specifically designed for patients with a goal INR of 2.0–3.0.

Frequency of Monitoring after Initiation

1. Flexible initiation method: INR daily through day 4, then within 3–5 days.
2. Average daily dosing method: INR within 3–5 days until INR above lower limit of therapeutic range, then within 1 week.
3. After hospital discharge:

   If stable: check INR within 3–5 days.

   If unstable: check INR within 1–3 days.
4. First month of therapy: check INR at least weekly.

Maintenance Therapy

This phase begins once the patient's INR is stable and a maintenance dose is established. It is important for the effectiveness and safety of warfarin that the INR remain within the therapeutic range. Routine monitoring of INR is required during warfarin therapy due to unexplained dose responses resulting from dietary changes, medication changes, poor compliance, comorbid diseases, or alcohol consumption.[8] See **Figure 5-1** for a patient assessment nomogram and **Table 5-4** for guidance on dosing adjustment during maintenance therapy.

Table 5-4. Dosing Adjustment during Maintenance Therapy

Goal INR 2.0–3.0	Recommended Action	Goal INR 2.5–3.5
<2.0	Reload x 0–1 Increase dose by 5–15%	<2.5
2.0–3.0	No change	2.5–3.5
3.1–3.5	Decrease dose by 0–15%	3.6–4.0
3.6–4.0	Hold 0–1 dose Decrease dose by 5–15%	4.1–4.5
>4.0	Hold dose until INR therapeutic +/– minidose vitamin K Decrease dose by 10–20%	>4.5

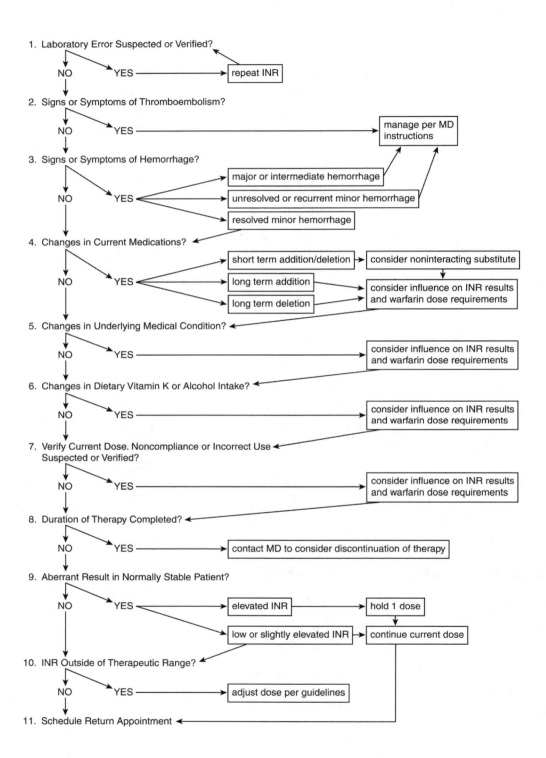

Figure 5-1. Patient Assessment

Frequency of Monitoring during Maintenance Therapy

1. If holding dose today in patient with significant over anticoagulation: check INR within 1–2 days.
2. If changing dose today: check INR within 1–2 weeks.
3. If dose change occurred <2 weeks ago: check INR within 2–4 weeks.
4. Routine follow-up for medically stable and reliable patients: check INR every 4 weeks.
5. Routine follow-up for medically unstable or unreliable patients: check INR every 1–2 weeks.

Guidelines for Correction of Over-Anticoagulation

Bleeding is the main complication of warfarin therapy. The risk of bleeding is associated with the intensity of warfarin therapy. Other variables that are associated with an increased risk of hemorrhagic complication are:

1. Age >65
2. Concomitant use of drugs that impair platelet function such as aspirin or nonsteroidal anti-inflammatory drugs (NSAIDs)
3. Co-morbid conditions such as renal insufficiency or anemia
4. History of gastrointestinal bleeding

The risk factors are additive and patients with two to three risk factors are at a significantly increased risk for bleeding.[8]

If the INR becomes supratherapeutic and the warfarin needs to be reversed, the recommendation is to administer oral vitamin K therapy and not intravenous (IV) or subcutaneous vitamin K. Oral vitamin K will quickly lower the INR but potentially not to a subtherapeutic range. Oral vitamin K will also prevent warfarin resistance once it is re-started compared to subcutaneous or IV vitamin K.[4]

See **Table 5-5** for recommendations for treating elevated INR.

Table 5-5. Management of Over-Anticoagulation

INR	Clinical Setting	Therapeutic Options
<5	Not bleeding	Hold warfarin until INR in range
5–9	Not bleeding	Hold warfarin until INR in range +/− minidose vitamin K orally 2.5 mg
>9	Not bleeding	Hold warfarin until INR in range and vitamin K 5–10 mg orally
Serious bleeding at any INR elevation	Rapid reversal required	Hold warfarin and vitamin K 1–10 mg slow IV infusion and repeat prn
Life-threatening bleeding	Rapid reversal required	Hold warfarin and give prothrombin complex concentrate with vitamin K 10 mg by slow IV infusion. Repeat prn

Peri-Procedural Anticoagulation

Management of an anticoagulated patient during a peri-operative period must be managed individually. For further assistance with risk assessment and recommendations on bridge therapy, see the Seventh American College of Chest Physicians (ACCP) Conference on Antithrombotic and Thrombolytic Therapy: Evidence-Based Guidelines[4] or University of Washington Medical Center Anticoagulation Services at www.uwmcacc.org.[11]

Drug Interactions and Herbal Information

Warfarin is metabolized by the cytochrome P450 system. Many drugs interact with warfarin through this mechanism, necessitating more frequent monitoring of the INR. A few interactions are significant enough to require close monitoring of the INR or a change in the warfarin dose once the interacting drug has been added. Another important factor to consider with any drug interaction is the timing of the two interacting drugs. For example, management is quite different if you are adding warfarin therapy to a patient on chronic therapy with an interacting drug as compared to adding an interacting drug to warfarin therapy. For complete drug interaction information, refer to *The Top 100 Drug Interactions: A Guide to Patient Management*.[12]

Many herbal products, including green tea, are becoming more popular and are often part of the patient's medications. Several herbal products interact with warfarin and may increase the risk of bleeding. Assessing herbal intake at each visit is an important facet of managing anticoagulation. For further information on interacting herbal products, see www.naturaldatabase.com or www.uwmcacc.org.[11]

Goals of Therapy

1. Safely and effectively manage thromboembolic disorders with anticoagulation therapy.
2. Ensure anticoagulation therapy is within the appropriate therapeutic range.
3. Minimize complications of antithrombotic therapy.
4. Prevent further thromboembolic events.

Clinical Pharmacy Goals

1. Identify patients who need antithrombotic therapy and assist the medical provider in the appropriate management of these patients.
2. Provide anticoagulation education and consultation to patients and medical staff.

Outcome Measures

Health outcome measures:

1. Incidence of major and minor hemorrhagic complications
    a. A major bleed classified as a hemorrhage, associated with:
        i.   A decrease in hemoglobin of at least 2 gm/dL
        ii. A transfusion of two or more units of red cells
        iii. Retroperitoneal or intracranial hemorrhage
        iv. Permanent discontinuation of the anticoagulant
        v.   Hospitalization
    b. Minor bleeding classified as a hemorrhage that did not meet the criteria for major bleeding.
2. Incidence of symptomatic recurrent thromboembolic events
3. Hospitalization due to recurrent thromboembolic events or hemorrhagic complications
4. Death due to thromboembolic or hemorrhagic causes

Patient Information Resources

1. Medline Plus: http://www.medlineplus.com
2. American Heart Association: http://www.americanheart.org
3. Coumadin: http://www.coumadin.com

CASE STUDY

S: Mr. IB is a 76-year-old male returning to clinic for anticoagulation follow-up. He was discharged from the hospital 5 days ago with atrial fibrillation. He was admitted for chest pain, dizziness, and increased heart rate. He states he had these symptoms for 7–10 days before going to the emergency room. He started on warfarin 2.5 mg daily and enoxaparin 80 mg subcutaneously q 12 h 6 days ago.

Problem list:

Uncontrolled hypertension

Atrial fibrillation

Type 2 diabetes

Benign prostatic hypertrophy (BPH)

Alcohol abuse (currently sober x 5 days)

He has several questions about warfarin and wants to know when he can stop the injections. He does not know why he is taking warfarin and was not given any patient education material at discharge. He denies any signs or symptoms (s/sx) of bleeding (nose bleeds, gum bleeding, blood in urine or stools) or bruising. He denies any lightheadedness, dizziness, weakness on one side, blurry vision, or chest pain. He does not feel his heart jumping around in his chest anymore and has more energy. He denies any alcohol use since discharge. Prior to that, he was drinking 6 beers daily with an extra pint of rum 1–2 times a week. Denies any other drug use.

Current medications:

Warfarin 2.5 mg daily x 6 days

Enoxaparin 80 mg subcutaneously q 12 h

Hydrochlorothiazide 25 mg daily

Lisinopril 40 mg daily

Metformin 1000 mg bid

NPH insulin 20 units at bedtime

Metoprolol SR 50 mg daily

ASA EC 81 mg daily

O:

INR   1.2 (goal 2–3)

BP   147/94

Pulse   82

Chem-7 and LFT all within normal range upon discharge from the hospital

A: INR subtherapeutic due to recent initiation of warfarin therapy 6 days ago at low dose. *Anticoagulation with warfarin is appropriate in this patient with atrial fibrillation due to high risk of stroke. Risk factors include age >65, hypertension, and diabetes.*[4]

P:

1. Increase warfarin dose to 5 mg daily. *This is the typical starting dose for the average daily dosing method as shown in Table 5-3.*

2. Stop enoxaparin since it is not indicated for atrial fibrillation. *Initial therapy with heparin or LMWH is indicated when thrombus is present and there is a high risk for embolism.*

3. Provide warfarin booklet and patient education material. Discuss s/sx of bleeding, bruising, and what to do if these occur. Discuss INR goal and risk of stroke if he decides not to be anticoagulated. Patient understands the need to be consistent with his diet and

activity and to report any changes. He understands the need to return to clinic (RTC) at least once every week until a maintenance dose is established. Reviewed what over-the-counter (OTC) products are safe to use with warfarin therapy.

4. Alcohol abuse. Encouraged patient to maintain his sobriety. Explained the risk of bleeding with alcohol use. Patient verbally stated he understands. He will continue to attend AA meetings 4–5 times weekly.

5. RTC in 3 days for INR and 1 week for cardiology appt.

References

1. American Heart Association. Heart disease and stroke statistics—2007 update. Available at http://www.americanheart.org/presenter.jhtml?identifier=1200026. Accessed April 16, 2007.

2. Deitcher SR. Antiplatelet, anticoagulant, and fibrinolytic therapy. In: Kasper DL, Fauci AS, Longo DL, et al., eds. *Harrison's principles of internal medicine*. 16th ed. New York, NY: The McGraw-Hill Companies, Inc; 2005:687–93.

3. Chiquette E, Amato MG, Bussey HI. Comparison of an anticoagulation clinic with usual medical care. *Arch Intern Med*. 1998; 158:1641–7.

4. Hirsh J, Albers GW, Guyatt GH, et al. The Seventh ACCP Conference on Antithrombotic and Thrombolytic Therapy: Evidence-Based Guidelines. *Chest*. 2004; 3(suppl):163S–703S.

5. Lovenox package insert. Bridgewater, NJ: Aventis Pharmaceuticals Inc.; November 2005.

6. Innohep package insert. Boulder, CO: Pharmion Corporation; January 2003.

7. Fragmin package insert. Kalamazoo, MI: Pharmacia and Upjohn Company; March 2004.

8. Hirsh J, Fuster V, Ansell J, et al. American Heart Association/American College of Cardiology Foundation Guide to Warfarin Therapy. *Circulation*. 2003; 107:1692–1711.

9. Harrison L, Johnston M, Massicotte P, et al. Comparison of 5 mg and 10 mg loading doses in initiation of warfarin therapy. *Ann Intern Med*. 1997; 126:133–6.

10. Crowther MA, Ginsberg JB, Kearon C, et al. A randomized trial comparing 5 mg and 10 mg warfarin loading doses. *Arch Intern Med*. 1999; 159:46–8.

11. University of Washington Anticoagulation Clinic Guidelines. Available at http://uwmcacc.org. Accessed November 1, 2006.

12. Hansten PD, Horn JR, eds. *The top 100 drug interactions: a guide to patient management*. Freeland, WA: H&H Publications; 2006.

Heart Failure

Steve Riddle

Heart failure (HF) is chronic and progressive, resulting in significant morbidity and mortality. HF affects about 5 million Americans and is responsible for substantial health care costs and resource utilization. It is a leading cause of hospitalization in people over the age of 65 and is estimated to be a contributing factor to nearly 250,000 deaths annually.[1] Clinical evidence demonstrates that pharmacologic therapies for HF can slow progression, decrease hospitalizations, and improve survival. Pharmacists are in an excellent position to assure early initiation and appropriate use of these valuable therapies for patients with HF.

Indications

Classification of HF

HF is differentiated based on ventricular function; filling defects are identified as diastolic HF, and pumping defects are noted as systolic HF. Most patients will either present with or progress to a condition that involves both aspects of ventricular dysfunction. Systolic dysfunction that results in a reduced ventricular ejection fraction (EF) plays a key role in determining appropriate pharmacotherapy.[2]

HF classifications have been developed to better understand the clinical status and disease progression in patients. The New York Heart Association (NYHA) functional classification gauges symptom severity over four phases (I–IV), while the American College of Cardiology and American Heart Association (ACC/AHA) system emphasizes the development and progression of HF over four stages (A–D).[2,3] While these classification approaches are significantly different, the intent is that they complement one another. **Table 6-1** provides a comparison of the two systems. The ACC/AHA classification is designed to match the stage of progression to the indicated evidence-based medication therapy and, therefore, may be the more useful tool for pharmacists.

Identification of HF Patients

In a collaborative practice setting, most patients with HF will be identified by a physician/provider and referred to the clinical pharmacist for appropriate management of medication-related therapies. Patients who present to the pharmacist with symptoms consistent with HF should be referred to the appropriate physician for complete diagnostic work-up.

It is important that health care providers identify patients with clinically evident HF and also those at risk for its development. Based on the ACC/AHA classifications, they are patients in Stage A and B who have no signs or symptoms of HF but have non-structural risk factors (e.g., hypertension, atherosclerotic disease, diabetes, obesity, family history of cardiomyopathy) or structural heart disease [e.g., previous myocardial infarction (MI), left ventricular (LV) remodeling, symptomatic valvular disease].[2]

Management

In addition to treating all patients with symptomatic HF, pharmacists should treat asymptomatic patients with moderately or severely reduced left-ventricular systolic function (EF <40%)—also known as Asymptomatic Left Ventricular Dysfunction (ALVD)—to slow or prevent progression to symptomatic HF.[4]

Lifestyle Recommendations

1. Regular exercise (mildly strenuous effort as tolerated) such as walking or cycling for all patients with stable HF.[2]

2. Dietary sodium restriction to 2–3 grams per day for all patients with HF. Patients with moderate to severe HF may require further restriction to <2 grams per day.[4]

3. Tobacco cessation should be encouraged and formally supported with counseling and medication therapy, as appropriate.

Pharmacologic Management

1. *ACE inhibitors (ACEIs).* ACEIs have a significant role in both prevention and treatment of HF. ACEIs are indicated in patients with known structural disease (Stage B) from ischemia without symptoms of HF or patients with systolic dysfunction. For patients with HF due to LV systolic dysfunction (EF <40%), therapy with an ACEI is supported by the highest level of evidence.[2] However, for patients in Stage A (at risk for HF), ACEIs have shown no advantage over other indicated therapies (e.g., antihypertensives) for preventing progression to HF.[2]

Table 6-1. Comparison of the NYHA and ACC/AHA Heart Failure Classification Systems*

ACC/AHA Stage		NYHA Functional Class	
Stage	**Description**	**Class**	**Description**
A	Patients at high risk of developing HF because of the presence of conditions that are strongly associated with the development of HF. Such patients have no identified structural or functional abnormalities of the pericardium, myocardium, or cardiac valves and have never shown signs or symptoms of HF.	No comparable functional class	
B	Patients who have developed structural heart disease that is strongly associated with the development of HF but who have never shown signs or symptoms of HF.	I(Mild)	No limitation of physical activity. Ordinary physical activity does not cause undue fatigue, palpitation, or dyspnea.
C	Patients who have current or prior symptoms of HF associated with underlying structural heart disease.	II(Mild)	Slight limitation of physical activity. Comfortable at rest, but ordinary physical activity results in fatigue, palpitation, or dyspnea.
		III(Moderate)	Marked limitation of physical activity. Comfortable at rest, but less than ordinary activity causes fatigue, palpitation, or dyspnea.
D	Patients with advanced structural heart disease and marked symptoms of HF at rest despite maximal medical therapy and who require specialized interventions.	IV(Severe)	Unable to carry out any physical activity without discomfort. Symptoms of cardiac insufficiency at rest. If any physical activity is undertaken, discomfort is increased.

*ACC/AHA = American College of Cardiology/American Heart Association; HF = heart failure; NYHA = New York Heart Association

2. *Beta blockers.* Beta blockers, along with ACEIs, form the foundation of pharmacotherapy for HF. Similar to ACEIs, beta blockers are indicated in all patients with known structural disease (Stage B) due to an ischemic event regardless of EF or presence of HF symptoms. Beta blockers are also indicated in patients with systolic dysfunction (EF <40%) and may be of increased benefit in patients with known coronary artery disease (CAD). All

patients with NYHA class II, III, or IV HF due to LV dysfunction should receive a beta blocker. Historically, use of beta blockers in patients with current or recent NYHA class IV symptoms has been controversial; however, evidence indicates that patients with more severe disease continue to benefit from these agents.[2]

Beta blockers are often used in conjunction with ACEIs. The goal is to titrate the beta blocker and ACEI to target doses as hemodynamic parameters allow. Because beta blockers are a heterogeneous class of agents, it is recommended that agent selection be limited to those agents with significant supporting clinical evidence and/or FDA approval for HF therapy. These agents include bisprolol, carvedilol, and extended-release metoprolol.

3. *Angiotensin II receptor antagonists or blockers (ARBs).* ARBs valsartan and candesartan have demonstrated beneficial outcomes in HF. Data from the CHARM-Added trial showed that adding candesartan to standard HF therapy, including an ACEI, provided both mortality and morbidity benefits.[5] However, other study results have been somewhat inconsistent, indicating that the agents do not yet possess the quantity of data attributed to ACEI. Therefore, ARBs can be considered for HF patients who suffer intolerable side effects with ACEI, or added to the HF regimen for patients receiving target doses of ACEI.

4. *Diuretics.* Diuretics provide no mortality benefit in HF; however, they are the only agents that can adequately and efficiently correct the edematous conditions that affect most HF patients. Therefore, patients with HF and signs of significant volume overload should receive diuretic therapy. The goal of diuretic therapy is to eliminate the clinical evidence of fluid retention. Combining diuretic therapy with the base HF therapies of an ACEI and a beta blocker, along with sodium restriction, can improve responsiveness to the diuretic and reduce the risk of clinical decompensation.[2]

Patients with mild volume overload may be managed on thiazide diuretics and, in patients with hypertension, this may confer a dual benefit. However, most HF patients and those with more severe volume overload will likely require a loop diuretic.[2]

It is important to note that response to diuretics may decrease with clinical progression of HF. Patients with persistent volume overload, despite initial medical management, may require alterations in their diuretic regimen, such as increased dose, use of a more potent diuretic, more frequent administration, and/or intravenous administration. First, consider any external factors impacting diuretic response, such as increased sodium intake or use of nonsteroidal anti-inflammatory drugs (NSAIDs). If a patient is unresponsive to high doses of diuretics and the options above have failed, resistance may be overcome through the use of a loop diuretic in combination with a thiazide diuretic. This combination prevents reabsorption of sodium at the distal tubule and can stimulate a profound diuresis. Use of these combinations, while clinically valuable, requires careful monitoring.

5. *Aldosterone antagonists.* Spironolactone has been shown to reduce mortality and hospitalization and improve functional class in patients with severe HF (NYHA class III with recent hospitalization or class IV symptoms) in patients on standard therapy (ACEI, loop diuretic, +/- digoxin).[6] This benefit is seen at low doses (12.5–25 mg/day), and is secondary to the agent's neurohormonal blockade (aldosterone-receptor antagonism) and not its diuretic effects. The indication for eplerenone is currently limited to HF post-MI infarction. The primary pharmacologic difference between these agents is a significant reduction of androgen-mediated side effects with eplerenone, most notably, gynecomastia. A practical, cost-effective approach to drug selection is to use spironolactone as a first-line agent with eplerenone reserved for patients who are intolerant to spironolactone.

Aldosterone antagonists should only be utilized in ".carefully selected patients with moderately severe or severe HF symptoms with recent decompensation or with LV dysfunction after MI."[2] Patients being evaluated for therapy with aldosterone antagonist should have a stable serum creatinine <2.5 mg/dL and a serum potassium <5.0 mEq/mL with no history of severe hyperkalemia. Also, it is recommended that these agents be given with loop diuretic therapy to minimize risk of hyperkalemia.[2,4]

6. *Digoxin.* Digoxin has demonstrated value in improving HF symptoms, quality of life, and exercise tolerance in patients with mild to moderate disease. There is also evidence that digoxin modestly decreased the risk of hospitalization in long-term (2–5 year) treatment of patients with NYHA Class II and III symptoms.[6] Because other agents are available that can improve the symptoms of HF while providing a known mortality benefit, digoxin is primarily recommended in patients who remain symptomatic after optimal management with ACEI, beta blockers, and/or ARB. Digoxin may be considered adjunctive therapy to beta blockers in patients with HF and atrial fibrillation.[2,5]

7. *Nitrates with hydralazine.* These agents have traditionally been considered a therapeutic option in patients who are intolerant of ACEI and ARB, or in patients with persistent symptoms after optimal doses of diuretics, ACEI, beta blockers, and digoxin. The utility of these agents has been questionable considering tolerability, dosing schedules, and increased pill burden.

More recently a large, randomized trial demonstrated a significant mortality benefit of this vasodilator combination in African Americans with HF, including those stabilized on ACEI.[8] The interpretation of this study for populations outside that studied is uncertain. However, as with all secondary therapies for HF that have demonstrated benefit, it is reasonable to evaluate a patient for addition of isosorbide and hydralazine if hemodynamics and other clinical parameters allow.[2,4]

8. *Medications contraindicated or not advised for use in HF*

   a. Class 1A (quinidine, procainamide, disopyramide) and Class 1C (flecainide, propafenone) anti-arrhythmic agents and sotalol increase the risk of death in patients with significant systolic dysfunction and are contraindicated.

   b. NSAIDs, including Cox-II selective inhibitors, are highly cautioned due to sodium and fluid retention and antagonism of diuretic therapy.

   c. Tricyclic antidepressants may cause cardiac arrhythmias.

   d. Thiazolidinediones (pioglitazone, rosiglitazone) may cause significant fluid retention.

Patient Monitoring and Follow-Up Evaluation

Careful history and physical examination should be the main guide to determining outcomes and directing therapy. Patients who have been hospitalized for HF should be seen or contacted within 1 week of discharge to make sure they are stable in the outpatient setting and to check their understanding of and compliance with the treatment plan. Since HF is a clinical syndrome as opposed to a primary diagnosis, numerous clinical features should be considered but most of them do not have defined goals or targets. Some basic parameters that pharmacists can monitor are noted below.

Objective Assessments

1. *Blood pressure (BP).* Blood pressure, sitting and standing, should be checked with each patient encounter to evaluate appropriate pressures and assess fluid status. Hypertension is a major cause and comorbidity of HF. Therefore, blood pressure goals (as established by the Joint National Congress on Hypertension) are <140/90 and ideally at the lowest pressures tolerated by the patient.[9] However, caution must be exercised to avoid hypotension, which may lead to cardiac decompensation and hemodynamic instability.

2. *Body weight.* A patient's weight is critical in assessing volume status. Establishing the person's euvolemic or "normal" weight allows comparisons over time and assists in HF monitoring. Unexplained weight gain >2–3 pounds in 1 day or 3–5 pounds in 5 days requires attention, especially if accompanied by significant worsening of cough, swelling, or shortness of breath.[4]

3. *Labs.* Electrolytes (especially potassium) and renal function should be included in routine HF monitoring.

Subjective Assessments

Subjective assessments for HF are primarily related to volume status and activity limitations. Clinicians should evaluate patients for signs of peripheral and pulmonary edema. Examples include presence of jugular venous distention (JVD); swelling of lower, dependent extremities; and significant worsening of cough or shortness of breath. Patients should also be evaluated for symptoms related to activity level (NYHA HF Classifications, Table 6-1).

Goals of Therapy

The universal goals of therapy for patients with HF include:

1. Reduce mortality

2. Improve quality of life

3. Maximize patient self-management

Medication-Related Goals

It is estimated that almost 50% of hospital admissions for HF are related to non-compliance with dietary instructions and/or medication use.[10] Pharmacists are in an excellent position to ensure success in achieving medication-related goals, which may include:

1. Initiation of evidence-based therapies

2. Appropriate monitoring of efficacy and safety

3. Assuring patient adherence and persistence with use of medications

4. Titration to medication dosages known to deliver or maximize therapeutic outcomes

   a. *ACE inhibitors (ACEIs)* (*with FDA-approved indications for HF or post-MI*)

ACEI	Initial Dose	Recommended Target Dose
Captopril	6.25–12.5 mg tid	50 mg tid*
Enalapril	2.5 mg daily or bid	10–20 mg bid*
Fosinopril	5–10 mg daily	20 mg daily
Lisinopril	5 mg daily	10–20 mg daily
Quinapril	5 mg bid	20 mg bid
Ramipril	2.5 mg bid	5 mg bid*
Trandolapril	1 mg daily	4 mg daily*

*Target dose established by clinical trials with reduced mortality as outcome.

   i. Once therapy is initiated, doses may be doubled every 3–7 days; the titration schedule may be more rapid or more slow, if clinically appropriate.

   ii. Following the initial dose of an ACEI in patients with HF, consider monitoring response for 2–3 hours or until BP is stabilized.

   iii. Lower initial doses of ACEI should be given if serum sodium is <135 mmol/L or in the presence of renal dysfunction (Scr >1.6 or Clcr <30 mL/min).

iv. Follow-up after initiation of therapy should be within 2 weeks and include reassessment of BP, electrolytes, and renal function.

b. *Beta blockers (with FDA-approved indications for HF)*

Beta Blocker	Initial Dose	Recommended/Target Dose
Bisoprolol	1.25 mg daily	5–10 mg daily
Carvedilol	3.125 mg bid	25 mg bid or 50 mg bid (if >85 kg)
Metoprolol XL	12.5 mg daily	100–200 mg XL daily

i. Once therapy is initiated, doses should be titrated as tolerated every 2–4 weeks to the target dose with careful monitoring of BP, heart rate, and fluid status.

ii. Patients should be advised that initiation of treatment and (to a lesser extent) dosage increases might be associated with transient symptoms of dizziness or lightheadedness (and rarely syncope) within the first hour after dosing.

iii. Episodes of dizziness or fluid retention during initiation can generally be managed without discontinuation of treatment and do not preclude subsequent successful titration or a favorable response.

c. *Angiotensin II receptor antagonists or blockers (ARBs)*

ARB	Initial Dose	Recommended/Target Dose
Candesartan	4 mg daily	32 mg daily
Valsartan	20–40 mg bid	80–160 mg bid

i. Once therapy is initiated, doses should be titrated up to the target dose as tolerated every 2 weeks with careful monitoring of BP, electrolytes, and renal function.

d. *Diuretics (This is not a complete listing of diuretics available in the United States.)*

Diuretic	Initial Dose*	Maintenance Dose*	Maximum Dose
Chlorthalidone	12.5–25 mg daily	50 mg daily	100 mg/24 hours
Hydrochlorothiazide	12.5–25 mg daily	25–50 mg daily	200 mg/24 hours
Bumetanide	0.5–1 mg daily	Titrate dose as needed	10 mg/24 hours
Furosemide	20–40 mg daily	Titrate dose as needed	600 mg/24 hours
Torsemide	10–20 mg daily	Titrate dose as needed	200 mg/24 hours

*Represents doses for chronic HF using oral agents and not acute treatment of severe volume overload. The appropriate dose of diuretic is highly dependent on patient need based on clinical status.

i. The goal of diuretic therapy is to eliminate fluid retention. In an ambulatory setting, doses of diuretics may be increased until urine output increases and weight decreases, generally by 0.5–1 kg daily.[2]

ii. Patients should be monitored closely when diuretic doses are being altered, especially with more aggressive regimens. Monitoring should include electrolytes, renal function, and hemodynamic parameters.

iii. Patients should keep records of their daily weights and bring those records when visiting their practitioners. Patients should be instructed to call their practitioners if they experience an unexplained weight gain >2–3 pounds in 1 day or 3–5 pounds in 5 days or significant worsening of cough, swelling, or shortness of breath. Instructing competent patients to self-titrate diuretic dosages to maintain proper fluid status is an excellent role for pharmacists and helps patients move towards self-management (**Appendix 6-1**).

e. *Aldosterone antagonist*

Aldosterone Antagonist	**Initial Dose**	**Recommended Dose**
Eplerenone	25 mg daily	50 mg daily
Spironolactone	12.5–25 mg daily	25 mg bid

i. Dose increase from the initial to recommended dose can be evaluated after 4 weeks of therapy. Dose adjustment based on potassium levels may be required.

ii. Potassium levels and renal function should be checked prior to and 3 and 7 days after initiation of therapy and then every month for 3 months. Once stable, monitoring should continue every 3 months.

iii. Supplemental potassium should generally be stopped, and patients should be educated on avoidance of high-potassium foods and NSAIDs.

iv. Patients with potassium levels >5.5 mEq/L should have the aldosterone antagonist discontinued or a significant dosage reduction, unless another cause for the hyperkalemia can be identified and corrected.

f. *Digoxin*

Dose: Therapy with digoxin should be initiated and maintained at a dose of 0.125–0.25·mg daily for most patients. In patients >70 years old, impaired renal function, or low lean body mass, a dose of 0.125 mg daily or every other day is recommended. At the recommended doses serum levels are not indicated, although these may be helpful in patients at risk for increased serum levels (e.g., renal impairment, drug interactions). The currently accepted range for digoxin plasma concentrations is 0.5–1 ng/mL.[2]

Monitoring: Ask patients about signs or symptoms associated with digoxin toxicity, such as gastrointestinal (e.g., nausea, anorexia) and neurologic (e.g., confusion, visual disturbances). If abnormal electrocardiogram

(ECG) readings are noted, digoxin toxicity should be considered a possible cause.

g. *Nitrates with hydralazine*

Dose: The target doses for this combination, used in the original V-HeFT clinical trial, were hydralazine 75 mg and isosorbide dinitrate 40 mg given qid. Patients were initiated at 50% of this dose on the qid schedule and then increased to the target dose at week two.[11] A more recent study, the African American Heart Failure Trial, used the product BiDil® (hydralazine 37.5 mg/isosorbide dinitrate 20 mg) with an initial dose of 1 tablet tid and titration to 2 tablets tid starting as soon as days 3–5.[8]

Monitoring: Check BP, volume status, and patient tolerability of medication.

Clinical Pharmacy Goals

1. Identify patients with or at risk for developing HF who are candidates for pharmacotherapy.

2. Create a pharmacotherapy care plan for HF that ensures evidence-based therapies are initiated appropriately and titrated to recommended doses.

3. Monitor patients within the appropriate timeframes for therapeutic response, tolerability, and safety parameters for all medications.

4. Insure adherence to and understanding of treatment plans for patients with HF and encourage patient self-management of condition based on ability level (**Appendix, Figure 6-1**).

Outcome Measures

The outcome measures below call for a numerator (number meeting outcomes indicator) and a denominator (total number qualifying or at risk for outcomes measure). For all the following outcome measures, consider pre/post intervention measurement comparisons. For example, baseline use of ACEI in patients with HF could be compared to the rate of ACEI use following targeted pharmacy/pharmacist efforts to improve utilization.

1. Care process measures

   a. ACEI therapy initiated (for qualifying patients without contraindications)

   b. Beta blocker therapy initiated (for qualifying patients without contraindications)

   c. Patients on both ACEI and beta blocker (for qualifying patients without contraindications)

   d. Patients provided with proper drug and disease management information (such as medication list with explanations, weight management chart with goals, dietary directions, and symptom management)

2. Surrogate clinical markers

   a. ACEI dose within target range (for all HF patients on ACEI therapy)

   b. Beta blocker dose within target range (for all HF patients on beta blocker therapy)

3. Health outcomes

   a. Hospitalization or readmission rates for HF-related causes

   b. Mortality rates for HF-related causes

   c. Improvement in exercise tolerance and ability to perform daily activities

Patient Information Resources

1. See Appendix, Figure 6-1 for Harborview Medical Center Self-Management Plan for Congestive Heart Failure

2. The Heart Failure Society of America: http://www.abouthf.org

3. The National Heart, Lung and Blood Institute (NHLBI): http://www.nhlbi.nih.gov/health/public/heart/index.htm

4. Medline Plus: http://www.nlm.nih.gov/medlineplus/heartfailure.html

5. American Heart Association: http://www.americanheart.org

CASE STUDY

S: DC is a 61 yo African American male who presents at clinic to establish care with a PCP. He is now referred to the pharmacist for pharmacotherapy management. DC is 4-weeks post-discharge from an urgent hospitalization, which resulted in a new diagnosis of HF. His hospitalization was characterized by an initial presentation of fluid overload with significant peripheral and pulmonary edema with complaints of nocturnal dyspnea and fatigue with routine activity. ECHO demonstrated an EF of 23% (AHA/ACC Stage 3 HF and NYHA Class II). He was aggressively treated with diuretics and initiated on an ACEI (and remained hemodynamically stable) and discharged on day 4.

DC reports no SOB or dyspnea in last 14 days and has been able to perform all usual daily tasks without fatigue, but does report he was quick to tire on recent 2-block walk up a moderate grade hill. He also denies any cough. He reports he has taken his medications as directed, although he cannot recall the names: "A new water pill and heart drug."

PMH:

1. Hypertension: diagnosed 10 years previous

2. MI (NSTEMI): 2 years previous

Family history: Father died at 50 yo in car accident. Mother is living and has hypertension. One sister (age 55y) with Type 2 diabetes mellitus.

Social/lifestyle: DC is divorced, lives alone, and has two children (both living out of state). DC denies history or current use of tobacco. Admits to occasional alcohol use (not excessive). He describes his activity level as low (minimal physical activity). His diet consists of three meals daily, composed primarily of fast food and processed foods.

Current medications:

Aspirin 81 mg daily (for 2 years)

Amlodipine 10 mg daily (for 4 years)

Enalapril 5 mg daily (started 4 weeks prior)

Furosemide 40 mg daily (started 4 weeks prior)

O: PE: No signs or symptoms of lower extremity edema; lung sounds normal on auscultation.

Labs:

Na 140	Scr 1.4	Chol (ttl) 190
Cl 108	BUN 18	LDL 120
K 4.6	HDL 30	
CO_2 26	Blood glucose (fasting) 92	

Vital signs:

BP (seated) 128/88   P 74

BP (standing) 132/90   P 70

Weight 78 kg (weight at recent hospital admission was 89 kg and 79 kg at discharge)

A/P:

1.   General: Patient with recent admission for newly diagnosed HF that is now clinically stable (NYHA Stage I Mild) but in need of refinement of medication therapy and initiation of evidence-based agents. Will alter medication regimen and begin patient education regarding management of HF. Follow-up appointment planned for 4 weeks in conjunction with PCP.

2.   *Patient appropriately started on ACEI therapy, enalapril 5 mg daily, for HF. Patient denies cough, episodes of dizziness, or other side effects. Electrolytes are normal (K = 4.6 on furosemide). Although some renal impairment is present, this is apparently stable with a Scr of 1.4 and normal fluid status.* Increase enalapril to 5 mg bid with planned increase to minimal target dose of 10 mg bid. Plan to recheck renal, hemodynamic, and electrolyte values at next visit. Review with patient rationale and appropriate use of ACEI and possible side effects.

3. *Patient's weight has decreased 11 kg from his hospital admission weight and appears euvolemic at a weight of 78 kg. It is unclear if therapy with a potent loop diuretic is necessary at this time. Initiation and dose titration of indicated neurohormonal therapies (ACEI, beta blocker) may negate the need for furosemide, as would improvements in dietary sodium restriction.* Decrease furosemide to 20 mg PO daily and evaluate at next visit for possible discontinuance. *Mild fluid retention may be treatable with HCTZ, which would provide added benefit for hypertension.* Discuss with DC the importance of weight as an indicator of fluid status and possible worsening of HF. Assure he has access to a scale and provide a system or tool that allows for daily weight monitoring. Instruct DC on use of the "stoplight" tool for interpreting weight changes and HF symptoms (including both fluid retention and dehydration) and when to seek medical attention. Discuss with DC the importance of dietary sodium restriction (2–3 grams/day). Explain that current diet likely contains foods that are very high in sodium. Refer DC to dietitian or provide educational information as appropriate.

4. *DC is indicated to receive beta blocker therapy. However, with upward titration of the enalapril and dose alterations with the furosemide, it may be prudent to initiate therapy at a future date.* Initiate low-dose metoprolol XL (12.5 mg daily) at the next visit as hemodynamic parameters allow. Consider delaying ACEI dose increase if necessary to allow for beta blocker.

5. CAD/post-MI: DC is considered at high risk for another CV event. *Aspirin is indicated. Patient reports no GI distress or evidence of GI bleed.* Continue aspirin at current dose.

6. Lipids: LDL is 120 and patient is high risk. LDL goal is <100 mg/dL. Initiate low-dose simvastatin at 10 mg QHS. Reevaluate in 8–12 weeks. Instruct patient on rationale for addition of agent.

7. Hypertension: Current BP is 132/90. Goal for DC is BP <140/90, although more optimal goal is 120/80. Patient is being treated with amlodipine 10 mg daily with recent addition of enalapril 5 mg daily. Discontinue amlodipine *as this agent has no proven morbidity or mortality benefit in HF.* Increase enalapril as planned with intent of adding beta blocker and titrating both agents to target dosages for HF. Reassess BP during this process. If further antihypertensive therapy becomes necessary, consider adding HCTZ. Discuss with DC the current blood pressure goals, the plans to achieve them, and the importance in doing so; especially in relation to HF. Assure he has access to BP monitoring and ask him to check BP twice weekly at a minimum and record values until the next appointment. Advise him to contact pharmacist or physician for BP >160/100. Encourage compliance with sodium restriction and advise on impact on blood pressure and HF.

8. Self-management: Patient states he is currently adherent to medications. Improvement is needed with diet and activity level. Provide complete medication list with clear directions for use and indications for each medication. Instruct on diet (as stated above). Encourage increase in activity level as tolerated and explain value of this for HF and overall cardiovascular health. Provide HF management tool (See Appendix, Figure 6-1) and basic disease information on HF.

References

1. Masoudi FA, Havranek EP, Krumholz HM. The burden of chronic congestive heart failure in older persons: magnitude and implications for policy and research. *Heart Fail Rev.* 2002; 7:9–16.

2. ACC/AHA 2005 guideline update for the diagnosis and management of chronic heart failure in the adult: a report of the American College of Cardiology/American Heart Association Task Force on Practice Guidelines (Writing Committee to update the 2001 Guidelines for the Evaluation and Management of Heart Failure). *Circulation.* 2005 Sep 20; 112(12):e154–235.

3. The Criteria Committee of the New York Heart Association. *Nomenclature and criteria for the diagnosis of the heart and great vessels,* 6th ed. Boston, MA: Little Brown and Co.; 1964.

4. Executive summary: HFSA 2006 comprehensive heart failure practice guideline. *J Cardiac Failure.* 2006; 12:10–38.

5. McMurray JJV, Ostergren J, Swederg K. Effects of candesartan in patients with chronic heart failure and reduced left-ventricular systolic function taking angiotensin converting-enzyme inhibitors: the CHARM-Added trial. *Lancet.* 2003; 362:767–71.

6. Pitt B, Zannad F, Remme WJ, et al. The effect of spironolactone on morbidity and mortality in patients with severe heart failure. Randomized Aldactone Evaluation Study Investigators. *N Engl J Med.* 1999; 341(10):709–17.

7. Digitalis Investigation Group. The effect of digoxin on mortality and morbidity in patients with heart failure. *N Engl J Med.* 1997; 336(8):525–33.

8. Taylor AL, Ziesche S, Yancy C, et al. Combination of isosorbide dinitrate and hydralazine in blacks with heart failure. *N Engl J Med.* 2004; 351:2049–57.

9. Chobanian AV, Bakris GL, Black HR, et al. The seventh report of the Joint National Committee for the Prevention, Detection, Evaluation and Treatment of High Blood Pressure (JNC 7 Report). *JAMA.* 2003; 289(19):2560–72.

10. Michalsen A, Konig G, Thimme W. Preventable causative factors leading to hospital admission with decompensated heart failure. *Heart.* 1998; 80:437–41.

11. Kohn G, Archibald DG, Ziesche S, et al. Effect of vasodilator therapy on mortality in chronic congestive heart failure. *N Engl J Med.* 1986; 314:1547–52.

Appendix 6-1: HMC Self-Management Plan for Congestive Heart Care

	Medications	Blood Pressure Screening	LDL-Cholesterol Test	Daily Weights	Low-Salt Diet	No Smoking
	Take all medications as prescribed.	At every office visit	Every 3–6 months	Take your weight each day.	Always. Low-salt diet is very important.	Smoking will increase your risk of a cardiac event 2–5 fold!
	• You should take an aspirin once a day unless allergic. • Your physician will prescribe other medications for your health needs. Ask your doctor or our pharmacist if you have questions.	Blood pressure control can reduce the risk of kidney failure, heart attacks, and stroke.	Cholesterol is an important controllable risk factor in coronary artery disease.	Weight gain over 2–3 lb/day or 3–5 lb in 5 days may be an alert to worsening congestive heart failure. Your Goal Weight _____	A diet that is ≤ 2 g of sodium and/or salt will decrease the retention of fluid and ease the work of the heart.	It is imperative that you stop smoking. For ways to help discontinue tobacco use, ask your physician.

Target Range	<130/80	<100	Stable Weight			
	Date/Result	Date/Result	Date/Result			
1st Quarter						
2nd Quarter						
3rd Quarter						
4th Quarter						

Appendix 6-1, Figure 6-1: HMC Self-Management Plan for Congestive Heart Care

Green Zone = All Clear

Your Weight = _____
- No shortness of breath
- No swelling
- No weight gain
- No decrease in your ability to maintain normal activity level

Green Zone Means:

- Your symptoms are under control
- Continue taking your medications
- Follow low-salt diet
- Keep physician appointments

Yellow Zone = "Caution"

If you have any of the following signs or symptoms:
- Increased weight >2–3 lb in 1 day or 3–5 lb in past 5 days)
- Increased cough
- Increased swelling
- Increased shortness of breath with activity
- Chest pain
- Increased number of pillows needed to sleep or need to sleep in a chair
- Anything else unusual that bothers you

Call your physician if you are in the YELLOW ZONE

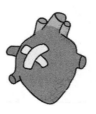

Yellow Zone Means:

- Your symptoms may indicate that you need an adjustment in your medications
- **Call your physician**

Primary Dr.: _____

Number: _____

RED ZONE = "Medical Alert"

- **Unrelieved shortness of breath**
- **Unrelieved chest pain**
- **Wheezing or chest tightness at rest**
- **Chest pain not relieved or recurs after taking Nitro tablets twice**

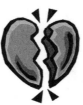

Red Zone Means:

This indicates that you need to be evaluated by a physician right away

Primary Dr.: _____

Number: _____

Cardiologist Dr.: _____

Number: _____

Asthma

Theresa O'Young

Asthma is a chronic inflammatory disease of the airways that affects over 20 million people in the United States.[1] Asthma is characterized by the classic triad of intermittent shortness of breath, cough, and wheezing. However, it is not unusual for one or more of these symptoms to be absent and fulfill the diagnosis of asthma. Mortality and hospitalization rates due to asthma exacerbations continue to increase in the United States, particularly among minority populations. Patients with asthma have more than 100 million days of restricted activities, reflected as days missed from work, school, and play.

The collaborative disease management model of practice provides an excellent mechanism to improve asthma care through a partnership with asthma patients. By improving techniques in medication delivery systems; educating patients about their disease state, medication therapy, and behavior modifications; and monitoring medication adherence, pharmacists can assist in significantly improving asthma outcomes.

Indications

Establish or confirm diagnosis by determining:

1. History or presence of episodic symptoms of airflow obstruction (e.g., wheezing, shortness of breath, chest tightness, or cough). Findings that increase the probability of the diagnosis of asthma include:

   a. Medical history: episodic wheezing; symptoms that worsen in the presence of allergens, irritants, or exercise; symptoms worsening at night; and patients with allergic rhinitis or atopic dermatitis.

b. Physical examination of the upper respiratory tract, chest, and skin that support the medical history. This includes inspection of the chest (noting skin color, temperature, and texture); palpation (feeling for tenderness, masses, and crepitation on the chest); and auscultation (listening for quality of breath sounds). Physical examination of the skin includes color, temperature, texture, and lesions.

2. Airflow obstruction that is at least partially reversible using spirometry.

3. Alternative diagnoses are excluded (e.g., vocal cord dysfunction, foreign bodies, other pulmonary diseases).

Management

1. A stepwise approach to drug therapy is used to gain and maintain control of asthma. Drug therapy includes long-term control and quick relief medications based on asthma severity (see **Table 7-1**[2]).

   a. Long-term control medications (controller medications)

      i. Inhaled corticosteroids provide long-term prevention of symptoms: suppression, control, and reversal of inflammation. Inhaled corticosteroid use also reduces the need for oral corticosteroids.

      ii. Oral corticosteroids are used for short-term burst therapy to obtain fast control of inadequately controlled persistent asthma.

      iii. Cromolyn sodium and nedocromil are mast cell stabilizers that provide long-term prevention of symptoms and may modify inflammation. This drug class can be used as preventative treatment prior to exercise or exposure to a known allergen.

      iv. Long-acting inhaled beta2-agonists are used for long-term prevention of symptoms, especially nocturnal symptoms. These agents are added to anti-inflammatory therapy and can also be used for prevention of exercise-induced bronchospasm.

      v. Methylxanthines can be used for long-term control or prevention of symptoms, especially nocturnal symptoms.

      vi. Leukotriene modifiers are used for long-term control and prevention of symptoms in mild persistent asthma.

   b. Quick-relief medications (rescue medications)

      i. Short-acting inhaled beta2-agonists are used for relief of acute symptoms. They can also be used as preventative treatment prior to exercise for exercise-induced bronchospasm.

      ii. Anticholinergics provide relief of acute bronchospasm in patients who may be using beta-blocker medications.

      iii. Oral corticosteroids are used for moderate to severe exacerbations

Table 7-1. Stepwise Approach for Managing Asthma in Adults and Children Over 5 Years Old

Classify Severity: Clinical Features Before Treatment or Adequate Control			Medications Required to Maintain Long-Term Control
	Symptoms/Day	PEF or FEV1	Daily Medications
	Symptoms/Night	PEF Variability	
STEP 4 Severe Persistent	Continual Frequent	Less than or equal to 60% >30%	**Preferred Treatment:** • High-dose inhaled corticosteroids AND • Long-acting inhaled beta$_2$-agonists AND, if needed: • Corticosteroid tablets or syrup long term (2 mg/kg/day, generally do not exceed 60 mg per day). (Make repeat attempts to reduce systemic corticosteroids and maintain control with high-dose inhaled corticosteroids.)
STEP 3 Moderate Persistent	Daily >1 night/week	>60% to <80% >30%	**Preferred Treatment:** • Low-to-medium dose inhaled corticosteroids and long-acting inhaled beta$_2$-agonists **Alternative Treatment** (listed alphabetically)**:** • Increase inhaled corticosteroids within medium-dose range OR • Low-to-medium dose inhaled corticosteroids and either leukotriene modifier or theophylline. If needed (particularly in patients with recurring severe exacerbations): **Preferred Treatment:** • Increase inhaled corticosteroids within medium-dose range and add long-acting inhaled beta$_2$-agonists **Alternative Treatment:** • Increase inhaled corticosteroids within medium-dose range and add either a leukotriene modifier or theophylline

continued on next page

Table 7-1. Stepwise Approach for Managing Asthma in Adults and Children Over 5 Years Old (cont'd)

Classify Severity: Clinical Features Before Treatment or Adequate Control			Medications Required to Maintain Long-Term Control
	Symptoms/Day	PEF or FEV1	Daily Medications
	Symptoms/Night	PEF Variability	
STEP 2 Mild Persistent	>2/week but <1x/day >2 nights/month	Greater than or equal to 80% 20–30%	**Preferred Treatment:** • Low-dose inhaled corticosteroids **Alternative Treatment** (listed alphabetically): • Cromolyn, leukotriene modifier, nedocromil, OR sustained-release theophylline to serum concentration of 5–15 mcg/mL
STEP 1 Mild Intermittent	Less than or equal to 2 days/week Less than or equal to 2 nights/month	Greater than or equal to 80% <20%	No daily medication needed Severe exacerbations may occur, separated by long periods of normal lung function and no symptoms. A course of systemic corticosteroids is recommended.

Step down: Review treatment every 1–6 months; a gradual stepwise reduction in treatment may be possible.

Step up: If control is not maintained, consider step up. First, review patient medication technique, adherence, and environmental control.

to prevent progression of exacerbations, reverse inflammation, speed recovery time, and reduce rate of relapse.

2. Asthma severity is classified according to symptoms reported by the patient. Initiate therapy at a higher level in the beginning to establish quick control, and then reduce the amount and frequency of medications. Continual monitoring is important to ensure that asthma control is achieved and maintained. Frequency and severity of symptoms to classify asthma severity can be determined by asking patients subjective questions, such as the following:

a. Are you able to sleep throughout the night without asthma symptoms?

b. Are you able to participate in normal activities of daily living without breathlessness?

c. Do you have the ability to walk, run, climb stairs, or carry packages up stairs without excessive shortness of breath or wheezing?

Objective information can be determined by a patient's recording of daily morning and evening peak expiratory flow rates, if the patient is using a peak flow monitoring device. Other useful data include the number of times per week that patients use their albuterol inhalers or other rescue medications.

3. Patient education begins at the time of diagnosis, and continues at each subsequent visit until goals and adequate understanding are achieved. Patient education may continue periodically as necessary thereafter. This should include:

   a. Defining asthma as a chronic lung disease characterized by inflammation of the airways. The patient should be able to list his or her symptoms and management goals.

   b. Discussing long-term care of asthma. Determining whether or not an action plan is appropriate. This is often developed collaboratively with the patient and clinician to provide the patient with directions on when symptoms signal additional treatment, or when further action is necessary.

   c. Discussing follow-up. Educating when and where the patient should call based on the severity of asthma symptoms:

      i. Clinic

      ii. Emergency department

      iii. 911 for medical assistance (e.g., if signs or symptoms of an asthma attack do not improve after 1 hour of using rescue medication every 20 minutes)

   d. Discussing expectations for asthma management and daily living. The ability to control asthma results in preventing chronic and troublesome symptoms, maintaining near normal lung function, maintaining normal activity levels (such as exercise or other physical activity), and preventing recurrent exacerbations.

   e. Discussing use of a peak flow meter for patient to monitor symptoms if appropriate. A peak flow meter should be recommended for patients who are interested in participating in objectively monitoring asthma symptoms.

   f. Education regarding the appropriate use of medications and devices:

      i. Use and purpose of rescue medications

      ii. Use and purpose of controller medications

      iii. Assessing inhaler technique and encouraging all patients to use a valved holding chamber or spacer

Goals of Therapy

1. Reduce inflammation, symptoms, and exacerbations.
2. Provide optimal pharmacotherapy agreed upon by the clinician and patient.

Pharmacotherapy should address the prevention of chronic and trouble-some symptoms as well as maintaining near normal pulmonary function and activity levels, including work attendance, exercise, and other physical activities. Pharmacotherapy should also be addressed to prevent recurrent exacerbations and minimize the need for emergency room visits or hospitalizations. It is also important to identify and minimize adverse effects from medications.

3. Identify and control factors contributing to asthma severity:

    a. Manage environmental triggers. Identify and appropriately treat or avoid allergens, occupational exposures, and environmental tobacco smoke.

    b. Rule out and treat other diagnoses that can potentially exacerbate asthma symptoms such as rhinitis, sinusitis, gastroesophageal reflux disease (GERD), viral respiratory infections, or medications (e.g., beta-blockers).

Clinical Pharmacy Goals

1. Identify patients needing drug therapy management

    a. Rescue medication use data: Patients utilizing albuterol or other rescue medications more than twice weekly may not be optimally treated according to stepwise approach to asthma management.

    b. Identify patients who are candidates for controller medications (based on the stepwise approach), but are not prescribed controller medications, or in whom doses of controller medications are suboptimal.

    c. Identify hospitalized patients or patients with emergency room visits as patients to target with medication therapy management.

2. Education

    a. Verify inhaler and peak flow technique.

    b. Ensure patients understand purpose and names of all prescribed asthma medications.

    c. Document patient education in the medical record.

Outcome Measures

1. Process measures: Decreased use of rescue medication; documented asthma action plan.

2. Health outcome measures: Reduction in emergency department visits and hospitalizations for asthma exacerbations.

Patient Information Resources

1. NHLBI: http://www.nhlbi.nih.gov/health/dci/Diseases/Asthma/Asthma_html
2. Asthma and Allergy Foundation of America: http://www.aafa.org
3. U.S. Environmental Protection Agency: http://www.epa.gov/asthma/ahop
4. American Lung Association: http://www.lungusa.org/site

CASE STUDY

S: SM, a 23-yo female, presents to clinic for an appointment with the pharmacist. Her primary care provider has referred her to the pharmacist to optimize drug therapy for asthma management and identify any other situations that might result in improved asthma control. She has been using her albuterol inhaler 3–4 times daily. When walking up stairs, she has to stop because of shortness of breath. She required a prednisone burst 1 year ago for an asthma exacerbation. She reports that she does have some wheezing, which gets better during the day but worsens at night. She is awakened at night with coughing at least 3 times a week. She reports having allergies to pollen and cats.

Past Medical History: Diagnosed with asthma when she was a teenager, 10 years ago.

Social History: Reports smoking socially, about ½-pack daily on the weekends.

Allergies: NKDA

Current medications:

Fenofexadine 60 mg bid

Albuterol 2 puffs qid prn shortness of breath

Fluticasone 220 mcg 2 puffs bid

Ortho-cyclen: 1 tablet daily

O: No pulmonary function tests in the last 10 years

A:

1. Asthma not optimally controlled as albuterol use is greater than twice weekly, and she is experiencing nighttime symptoms more than 1 night per week.

2. Smoking cessation and allergy management will contribute to improving asthma control.

3. Controller medications for asthma control can be optimized.

P:

1. Assess readiness to quit smoking and refer to appropriate smoking cessation assistance as needed.

2. Review allergy control; recommend nasal steroids if needed.

3. Review inhaler technique; provide valved holding chamber or spacer as needed.

4. Recommend peak flow monitoring and instruct patient on use of information.

5. Recommend addition of long-acting beta agonist for long-term control.

6. Review patient's environment for other triggers specific to home as symptoms worsen at night.

7. Review patient's medical condition for post nasal drip and/or GERD that might contribute to nighttime coughing.

8. Plan follow up for 6–8 weeks with pharmacist.

References

1. American Lung Association. Asthma in adults fact sheet. Available at http://www.lungusa.org/site/pp.asp?c=dvLUK9O0E&b=22596. Accessed April 18, 2007.

2. NHLBI Expert Panel 2: Guidelines for the Diagnosis and Management of Asthma. June 2002.

Tobacco Cessation

Steve Riddle

Tobacco use remains the nation's leading preventable cause of premature death. Data from the Centers for Disease Control and Prevention (CDC) collected from 1995 to 1999 estimates that more than 440,000 Americans die annually from disease caused by tobacco use.[1] Cigarette smoking is solely responsible for more than 30% of cancer deaths in the United States each year.[1] Smoking also contributes to heart disease, stroke, and chronic obstructive pulmonary disease. Although overall rates for cigarette smoking have trended down in recent years, 44.5 million or 21% of U.S. adults still smoke.[2] An estimated 3.75 million or 22% of U.S. high school students report regular use of tobacco.[2] The impact of tobacco use on society is enormous. From 1995 to 1999, annual costs in the United States were assessed at $75.5 billion for direct medical care and $81.9 billion for lost productivity.[1]

All health care professionals share a responsibility to discourage the initial and continued use of tobacco products. Pharmacists, as highly trusted and accessible health care providers, are in a unique position to inform, educate, and assist patients who want to quit smoking or using tobacco.

Indications

Identifying Smokers and Tobacco Users

Screening questions regarding tobacco use must be incorporated into the usual processes of medical care—at every admission and discharge and at every clinic visit. The goal should be not only to determine tobacco use, but also to evaluate the patient's interest in quitting.

Several tools and guidelines are beneficial in developing tobacco use screening and assessment programs. The Surgeon General and Public Health Guide, Treating Tobacco Use and Dependence, recommends the 5 A's and 5 R's tools. The 5 A's—Ask, Advise, Assess, Assist, and Arrange—correspond to the five critical steps in building a successful, systematic approach to cessation efforts. The 5 R's are designed to motivate smokers currently not interested in quitting by determining relevance, risks, rewards, roadblocks, and repetition to quitting. Information is available at http://www.surgeongeneral.gov/tobacco/clinpack.html.

The following is an example of a screening tool developed at our institution for identifying tobacco users and determining readiness to quit (RTQ) status. The tool is an abbreviated version of the 5 A's.

TOBACCO USE IDENTIFICATION AND RTQ TOOL

1. "Have you ever smoked or used tobacco products?"

   ❑ Never

   ❑ Former

   ❑ Current ⇒ If current, move to question #2

2. "Are you interested in quitting within the next 30 days?"

   ❑ No ⇒ Give strong quit message and inform about cessation resources available

   ❑ Yes ⇒ Give strong quit message and refer to counseling

Determining Interest in Quitting

The Transtheoretical Model (TTM) is a common method for classifying a smoker's interest in quitting. It describes six distinct stages that people move through when making significant cognitive and behavioral changes. This model, developed by Prochaska and DiClemente in 1983, has been successfully applied to numerous health risk behaviors.[3] The six stages of TTM include the following:

1. Precontemplative: Not ready to make changes at this time.

2. Contemplative: Ambivalent about the value of changing versus not changing.

3. Preparation: Ready to make a change.

4. Action: In process of making changes.

5. Maintenance: Has successfully made lasting changes.

6. Relapse: Lasting change attempts were unsuccessful, and previous behavior has resumed.

Awareness of the patient's current stage supplies critical information to providers involved in tobacco cessation counseling. The RTQ tool assists by asking if the patient is ready to quit within the next 30 days. A "yes" indicates the person is in the preparation stage and ready to take action in a short, defined period of time. It is estimated that 20% of all smokers are in the preparation stage.[4] These patients should be referred to formal smoking cessation counseling. Smokers in earlier stages should receive information and support that helps them advance towards the preparation stage.

Management

Once a smoker has decided he or she is ready to quit, efforts can be made to analyze the level of addiction and dependence. While DSM-IV official diagnostic criteria are available for nicotine dependence and withdrawal (305.1, 292.0),[5] they are not particularly helpful in clinical practice. One of the most commonly used tools for assessing smokers is the Test for Nicotine Dependence.[6] This tool rates a smoker's dependence on nicotine using six questions with a cumulative point total from 0–10; a score of 8–10 indicates very high dependence.

Another tool for both patient and counselor education is the tobacco addiction pie, developed at our institution (**Figure 8-1**). The pie helps visualize the key aspects of tobacco addiction: physical, psychological, behavioral, emotional, and social. Pharmacists are familiar with physical dependence to nicotine and understand most users will experience withdrawal symptoms upon quitting. However, many pharmacists are not as familiar with the other aspects of tobacco addiction. Not all smokers will have each slice of the pie, but most will have several components.

While tobacco addiction is complicated and each patient will have unique needs, two strategies are commonly used in cessation counseling. They are pharmacologic and non-pharmacologic (e.g., cognitive–behavioral therapy).

Non-Pharmacologic Strategies for Tobacco Cessation

Smokers sometimes attempt to quit by using alternative methods such as hypnosis, acupuncture, and dietary supplements. Although indi-

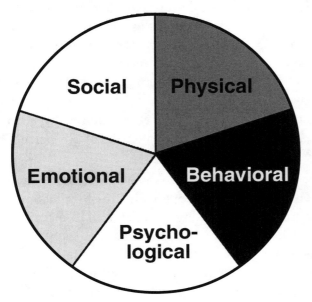

Figure 8-1. Tobacco Addiction Pie: Aspects of Addiction

viduals may have success, no data support these or other highly advertised smoking "cures."

Cold turkey cessation attempts are characterized by a sudden stopping of tobacco use or nicotine intake with no cessation counseling or medication support. Success rates with this approach average around 2–5% (compared to 10–20% for those using formal cessation services with medications).[7] Some smokers use tapering as a method to gradually decrease nicotine intake. Tapering is challenging and quit rates are similar to cold turkey, but this approach may be helpful in decreasing cigarette use prior to a planned cessation attempt for those with heavy smoking habits.

The best evidence-supported, non-pharmacologic approach to quitting involves cognitive–behavioral therapy.[8] A key component of tobacco addiction is behavioral. When interviewing smokers, it is important to ask about what triggers the desire for a cigarette. Routinely, smokers will link smoking with certain activities such as eating, driving, drinking coffee, work breaks, and talking on the telephone. For most patients, smoking has become so linked to this other activity that it is an unconscious habit to do both simultaneously. The first step in addressing these triggers is to increase awareness. Ask smokers to list typical times and situations during which they normally smoke. Prompt them with examples. Encourage them to continue to think about routines and tasks they are engaged in when they smoke. Tell them to be aware of when they experience a craving or urge to smoke.

Behavioral modification involves several strategies. One approach is to substitute a new behavior in place of the old. If the person has a cigarette after dinner, consider advising substitution of a snack or light dessert. Another strategy is to change the situation or environment. If the cigarette was usually smoked at the table, then suggest the person move into a new location or situation. Replacing a bad habit with a good habit is always the best strategy. Advise the patient to go for a walk or engage in some form of exercise in place of the previous routine. Many smokers watch TV and smoke. Avoiding this situation, at least during the early quit attempt period, may be helpful. Also, changing the area around the TV, such as rearranging furniture or sitting in a different place, can alter the brain's perception of the environment and may diminish the trigger.

It is well documented that many tobacco users have some underlying anxiety and/or depression.[9] Smokers often use nicotine to cope with stressful situations. Nicotine can invoke euphoria and provide a calming effect as well as increased concentration and the ability to focus. Severe or stressful situations, such as the death of a family member or loss of a job, are commonly implicated in relapses. Not all emotional triggers are negative. Cigarettes can be used to celebrate a special occasion or as a reward (e.g., at the end of a hard day's work). In these cases, smokers have learned to cope with or enhance an experience using tobacco. If the cessation strategy does not include ideas or methods for dealing with these situations, then slips and relapses are likely. Therefore, it is critical to develop strategies for dealing with the emotional triggers, such as relaxation techniques (e.g., deep breathing, relaxing music), building social support, and finding healthy rewards to replace cigarettes. For cases of clinically significant anxiety or depression, referral to an appropriate medical provider is warranted.

Some smokers may feel that the cigarette does something for them that they are unable to do themselves. For example, smokers may say, "cigarettes help in dealing with stress and staying calm," or "they help control weight." In this sense, smokers become psychologically dependent on the cigarette. It is critical then to give them other strategies to demonstrate that they, not the cigarette, are in control.

Social aspects of smoking are important to consider. Smokers may define themselves by their social groups and status. Often a smoker's social circle may contain many smokers, which makes quitting even more difficult. Avoiding this group may leave the smoker isolated at a time when social support is critical. Smokers need to develop strategies for socializing (e.g., escape plans for trigger situations), connecting to cessation support groups (e.g., local meetings, Internet chat rooms), and diminishing risky situations.

Pharmacologic Strategies for Tobacco Cessation

Several agents have been studied for efficacy in tobacco cessation, including the prescription agents nortriptyline and clonidine. Many have shown little or no effectiveness in helping patients maintain prolonged abstinence (6 or 12 months tobacco-free).[10]

Nicotine Replacement Therapy

Nicotine replacement therapy (NRT) has been reported to almost double cessation rates compared with placebo, regardless of other supportive interventions.[11] Despite considerable differences in kinetics, duration of action, routes of administration, and adverse effects among the various nicotine preparations, overall efficacy is approximately the same.[11] Therefore, selection from the various NRT products will depend on patient-specific considerations such as personal preference, experiences with previous cessation therapies, ability to titrate dose, and tolerability (**Table 8-1**).

Since NRTs are based on smoking rates of up to 20–25 cigarettes a day, smokers whose daily consumption exceeds these rates may require higher initial doses of NRT to prevent withdrawal symptoms and cravings. High-dose NRT has been explored in several studies. Combinations of NRT, generally the patch and a titratable product such as the gum or lozenge, have been shown to be more effective than a single agent.[11] However, there are no safety data regarding these NRT combinations. One study by Shiffman et al. demonstrated the efficacy of using 35 mg nicotine per 24 hours via transdermal patch in the first 3 days of a cessation attempt.[12]

Table 8-1. Nicotine Replacement Products

NRT Product	Dosing	Considerations for Use
Nicotine Gum 2 mg, 4 mg	If >25 cigarettes/day, use 4 mg. If ≤25 cigarettes/day, use 2 mg. Chew one piece q 1–2 hours initially for 1–6 weeks, then taper by 50% q 2 weeks. Typical duration of use is 8–12 weeks.	• Not a suitable product for those with poor dentition or jaw problems. • GI side effects can be problematic. • Requires proper chewing technique. • May satisfy oral cravings. • Patients can titrate therapy.
Nicotine Patch 7 mg, 14 mg, 21 mg (the most common product strengths)	If ≥10 cigarettes/day, initiate with 21-mg patch. If <10 cigarettes/day, initiate with 14-mg patch. Maintain initial patch for 4–6 weeks and then taper q 2 weeks to 7-mg patch. Typical duration of use is 8–10 weeks.	• Dermatalogic conditions or allergic reactions may prevent use. • Ease of use may improve compliance. • Cannot titrate dose.
Nicotine Lozenge 2 mg, 4 mg	If >25 cigarettes/day, use 4 mg. If ≤25 cigarettes/day, use 2 mg. Use 1 lozenge q 1–2 hours initially for 1–6 weeks, and then taper by 50% q 2 weeks. Typical duration of use is 8–12 weeks.	• GI side effects can be problematic. • May satisfy oral cravings. • Patients can titrate therapy. • Oral alternative to gum, especially for patients with dentition and jaw problems.
Nicotine Nasal Spray	1–2 doses/hour (8–40 doses/day). *Note*: 1 dose = 2 sprays (one in each nostril). Max dose: 5/hr or 40/day Recommended period of use is 3–6 months with gradual reduction. Patients should not inhale, but passively spray into nares.	• Nasal and throat irritation, cough, and tearing can be problematic. • Not recommended for patients with nasal disorders or severe reactive airway disease. • Patients can titrate therapy.
Oral Nicotine Inhaler	Recommended range: 6–16 cartridges/day. Cartridges provide for 20 minutes of continuous puffing. Inhalation should target the back of the throat, not the lungs. Recommended use is 3–6 months with gradual reduction.	• Nasal and throat irritation can be problematic. • Unpleasant taste. • Patients can titrate therapy. • Closely mimics smoking hand-to-mouth behavior. (Pro or con?) • Caution recommended for patients with bronchospastic disease.

Bupropion

Bupropion approximately doubles cessation rates relative to placebo, and studies have demonstrated rates significantly higher than with the nicotine patch.[13] Therapy should be initiated at least 1 and ideally 2 weeks before the cessation date at a dose of 150 mg per day for 3 days. Then the dose should be increased to 300 mg per day. Duration of therapy should be at least 7–12 weeks but may be continued for up to 6 months. Quick titration aids in avoiding side effects such as insomnia, nervous system problems (e.g., tremors), and dry mouth. Patients experiencing insomnia may benefit from taking their second daily dose in the afternoon (at least 8 hours after the first daily dose).

Bupropion may be the preferred therapy in patients with underlying mood disorders (e.g., depression), at risk for significant cessation-related weight gain, or with a history of failed cessation attempts with NRT. Patients with a history of or at risk for seizures, anorexia, or bulimia are not suitable candidates for bupropion.

Varenicline

Varenicline is the medication most recently approved for cessation. A highly selective alpha-4, beta-2, nicotinic acetylcholine receptor partial agonist, varenicline has shown superior efficacy versus placebo in several trials and from similar to superior efficacy to bupropion in another trial.[14] Following the recommended 7-day titration, the maintenance dose of varenicline for cessation is 1 mg twice daily. The most common adverse effect noted in clinical trials was nausea, occurring at rates of around 30% with discontinuance rates approaching 3%.[15]

Combination Therapies

All the above-mentioned drugs and products are approved for single-agent therapy; however, combinations may be useful for patients who are unable to quit with monotherapy alone.[16] Theoretically, combining bupropion with NRT may provide the best clinical advantage since the agents have varying mechanisms of action. Also less data support appropriate nicotine dosing when combining NRT formulations.

Selecting a Cessation Medication

No evidence-based guidelines or algorithms assist in determining the best choice of cessation medication for an individual patient. Our organizational approach is to present cessation medication options and allow patients to direct which therapy or combination is of most interest to them. The counselors gather specific information on previous cessation therapies, response to these therapies, current medications, and significant medical history and then provide input for consideration in agent selection. Although selection of an effective agent is important, it is even more important to select one that is least likely to contribute to a negative outcome.

Bupropion has the potential for many drug–drug and drug–disease interactions. Similarly, patients with known skin reactions to adhesives may not tolerate the nicotine patches, and patients with poor dentition may not be good candidates for nicotine gum. One key consideration is patient control of nicotine intake; nicotine gum, inhaler, nasal spray, and lozenge products allow patients to assert more active control. Patches allow less control, but are more suitable for patients who don't wish to actively manage their nicotine intake.

Appointments and Monitoring

In developing a tobacco cessation program, you should determine the visit method. Options include individual (one-on-one) appointments, group classes, and telephone visits. This determination should be based on available resources, ease of access and appointment scheduling for patients, and the size of the program. From an evidence-based standpoint, more data support direct contact with patients and development of a rapport between the counselor and patient (see "Clinical Pharmacy Goals").[9]

In our organization, group classes serve as our primary means of providing cessation services. These classes provide built-in social support and include a brief one-on-one opportunity for counselors to assist in developing personalized quit plans. For patients who cannot attend group sessions, one-on-one appointments are available with pharmacists in the primary care clinics.

Because the goal of tobacco cessation is abstinence, a key focus during follow-up is a status check on tobacco use. It is important to ask about slips and relapses. Relapses indicate reversion back to the previous behavior. A relapse can be viewed as a time when the patient needs to reevaluate his or her interest in quitting. Motivation, confidence, and persistence are crucial ingredients for a successful quit attempt and may be diminished immediately following a relapse. A brief period of reflection to reenergize for the next attempt may be beneficial for some patients. At our institution, whenever a patient wishes to make another cessation attempt, he or she should be asked to (re)enroll in the initiation class. Cessation literature indicates that most people will quit and relapse multiple times prior to a successful attempt.[17]

Slips refer to isolated incidences of smoking (usually just one or two cigarettes) and a return to abstinence. Slips should be taken seriously as many smokers relapse with just one incidence. While it is normal (and probably appropriate) that smokers feel guilty about a slip, it is important to instruct the person to view this as a learning opportunity. Slips often provide information regarding triggers, such as stressful situations or problematic social or environmental events. In addition to triggers, look for barriers that may prevent people from moving forward. For example, weight gain can be a significant problem for some cessation patients. Discussing a variety of strategies in dealing with this barrier (e.g., healthy snacks, drinking water, stress reduction for nervous eaters, increasing exercise) is an excellent approach.

Drug therapy and general cessation progress must be monitored. Follow-up with patients should occur at a minimum of every 2 weeks. Specific questions should be asked regarding the frequency and intensity of cravings, the occurrence of any slips (if any), success in applying non-pharmacologic interventions, and any possible adverse or undesirable reactions to cessation medications. Adjustments are made accordingly. The duration for most cessation therapy is 8–12 weeks. However, it is useful to focus more intently on the continual progress of the patient towards the ultimate goal of tobacco abstinence. If a patient is making continual progress and shows commitment to quitting, then longer treatment durations may be acceptable.

Goals of Therapy

1. Pharmacist assistance in helping patient achieve sustained abstinence from tobacco.
2. Patient adherence to and appropriate use of cessation medications.
3. Patient compliance with appointment/visit schedules.

Clinical Pharmacy Goals

Identification of tobacco users and assessment of their interests in quitting should be goals for all health professionals and health systems. Pharmacists must consider the provision of appropriate cessation medications based on patient needs, current medications, and other health conditions. From a broader perspective, current data indicate that a counseling program should address the following five criteria in order to achieve optimal outcomes:[17]

1. Ensure the provider has an appropriate level of training.
2. Provide ≥4 sessions lasting at least 10 minutes using evidence-based guidelines.
3. Deliver a total, cumulative contact time of >30 minutes.
4. Ensure sessions take place over at least 2 weeks, preferably 8 weeks or more.
5. Ensure the tobacco users are well informed and educated about the various medications available.

Outcome Measures

The Joint Commission requires hospitals to collect data regarding tobacco cessation screening and provision of cessation advice and counseling for several diagnoses (heart failure, acute myocardial infarction, pneumonia). Key process measures state that (1) patients are asked about tobacco status; (2) tobacco users are provided tobacco cessation advice or counseling; and (3) both of the aforementioned measures are documented. It is highly recommended that these metrics are in place for all patients in the inpatient and ambulatory setting. An initial target should include high-risk patients (e.g., COPD) or specific populations (e.g., primary care clinic). Goals should be 100% compliance for all measures.

Provision of more formal tobacco cessation counseling warrants the capture of specific data in order to track and demonstrate outcomes. A Microsoft® Access™ database provides a convenient method to capture key data. Pertinent information includes patient clinical indicators (tobacco use types, rate, pack years, current status), cessation medication provided (e.g., NRT, bupropion), appointment data (number of appointments per patient, number of total visits per month), adverse reactions to cessation therapy, and cessation counseling outcomes.

The goal of tobacco cessation is long-term abstinence, although it is difficult to monitor. Most clinical literature examines 3-, 6-, and 12-month periods of tobacco abstinence, which is also challenging to track. Therefore, it is advisable that other care and process measures be included among the quality metrics in addition to abstinence. Examples of other measures to consider include total number of patients who are seen, total visits, number of visits per patient, total receiving pharmacotherapy, and number or percent completing program.

Resources

Provider Resources

Two types of cessation training programs are available. Short programs (1–2 hours) are designed to assist health care workers in performing tobacco use screening and brief interventions (i.e., the 5A's). More intense cessation interventions are handled in longer programs (in excess of 8 hours). One program designed specifically for pharmacists is available from Rx for Change at no cost (http://rxforchange.ucsf.edu/). Developed at the University of California, San Francisco, it allows the download of PowerPoint presentations, clinical tools, and patient education information that is helpful in developing an internal training program. Another resource is the Pharmacy Partnership for Tobacco Cessation. This group is organizing a national repository of education tools, resources, and training assistance options for cessation. Information and materials are available at www.ashp.org by clicking on "Resource Centers" and then on "Tobacco Cessation." Other resources include the local public health department, the local American Lung Association chapter, and the American Cancer Society.

Patient Information Resources

Patient information resources for tobacco cessation are plentiful. Local and state agencies and organizations are excellent resources for materials and social support groups. See **Table 8-2** for a partial list of resources available in the United States.

Table 8-2. Tobacco Cessation Resources

Source	Contact Info	Comments
Agency for Healthcare Research and Quality (AHRQ)	www.ahcpr.gov	Information for providers and patients. The definitive source for guidelines, data, systems design, etc.
American Lung Association	www.lungusa.org	Programs, materials, and miscellaneous information.
American Lung Association, Washington	www.alaw.org 1-800-732-9339	Patient information, posters.
American Cancer Society (NW division)	www.cancer.org 1-800-ACS-2345	Patient information, posters, reports, statistics, etc. Search under "tobacco."
American Heart Association	www.americanheart.org 1-800-242-8721	Smoking and heart disease brochures for patients.
National Cancer Institute	1-800-4-CANCER	Cessation brochures and information for patients. In English and Spanish.
U.S. Surgeon General	www.surgeongeneral.gov/tobacco	Tobacco Dependence Guidelines and some patient information.
Quit Net	www.quitnet.com	On-line: patient information, counselors, social support group, EBM quit info. In Spanish and English.
Freedom From Smoking (ALA)	www.ffsonline.org	An on-line quit smoking program for tobacco users.
Why Quit?	www.whyquit.org	A great site for patient education, introspection, and assistance. *Note*: they support only a cold turkey, no-medication approach to quitting.
Nicotine Anonymous	www.nicotineanonymous.org	12-step program, patient information, group chat-line support. *Caution*: tied to a fair amount of product advertisement.
Nicotrol Helping Hand	www.helpinghand.com	An on-line smoking cessation program for tobacco users. Sponsored by Pfizer.

continued on next page

Table 8-2. Tobacco Cessation Resources (cont'd)

Source	Contact Info	Comments
Tobacco Free Kids	www.tobaccofreekids.org	Website that focuses on the health risks of smoking from a social–political perspective.
Pharmacia	1-877-872-8535 (Pharmaceutical Co.)	Free Nicotrol inhalers and quit kits.
GlaxoSmithKline	1-800-496-3772, ext 8297	Nicoderm (patches), Nicorette (gum), lozenges can be obtained for qualified providers/patients. Zyban available to providers. Need form to request products. Quit kits are also available.
Boehringer Ingelheim Pharmaceuticals	1-877-933-4310, ext 9443	Smoking cessation patient education materials.
Tobacco Prevention Resource Center	seattle@jba-cht-com 206-447-9538 Fax 206-447-9539	Tobacco cessation training for health care providers. Also, training and education for community groups.
Quit Smoking Support Resource	www.quitsmokingsupport.com	Comprehensive, on-line support service for adults.
CDC Site for Tobacco Prevention & Control	www.cdc.gov/tobacco/	Links to reports and statistics on smoking, especially for high-risk groups.
National Quitline (via HHS)	www.smokefree.gov 1-800-QUITNOW	Phone contact puts users in touch with programs that can help them give up tobacco. Website offers live online advice during specific hours and information to make cessation easier.
Smoke Free Families	www.smokefreefamilies.org	Website with focus on pregnancy and smoking. Information for health care workers and lay persons.

CASE STUDY

S: SJ is a 54 yo male with recent hospitalization for exacerbation of COPD who presents at clinic for tobacco cessation counseling. SJ reports increased displeasure with smoking over the last year and an interest in quitting as soon as possible to preserve his health. He reports increased coughing episodes and shortness of breath with moderate activity in the last year. He describes two previous attempts to quit smoking, the most recent being 3 years ago with an abstinence period of 6 weeks. No cessation medications were used in either attempt. Patient interview discovers major triggers that include morning routines, coffee, post-meals, and stressful situations. SJ indicates an interest in using NRT with a preference for patch vs. gum due to dental problems.

PMH: Significant for head injury (S/P 8 years) with pursuant seizure disorder treated with phenytoin. Last recorded seizure was 6 years ago. Anticonvulsant therapy was discontinued 5 years ago. BPH (diagnosed 2 years ago).

Allergies: Penicillin (anaphylaxis)

Current medications:

Tiotropium Inhaler 1 puff daily

Salmeterol Inhaler 2 puffs twice daily

Albuterol MDI 2 puffs every 6 hours as needed

Terasozin 2 mg q hs for BPH

Aspirin 325 mg daily for cardioprotection

O: Vital signs BP 152/88, Pulse 74, Wt 72 kg

Currently smokes approximately 1.25 packs per day (25 cigarettes)

Fagerstrom Score = 7 (indicating high dependence on nicotine)

A/P: Patient in preparation stage for tobacco cessation and indicates readiness to initiate attempt at soonest possible date.

1. Create list of smoking triggers and have patient develop initial action plan for each, including cognitive/behavioral and emotional coping strategies. Management of cravings is reviewed.

2. Initiate pharmacotherapy with nicotine transdermal patch at 21 mg per day based on current cigarette consumption. Initial plan is for 6 weeks at the 21-mg patch strength followed by 14 mg for 2 weeks and 7 mg for 2 weeks with possible alterations depending on progress. SJ is instructed in appropriate patch use, possible side effects, and goals of NRT therapy. He is also educated regarding nicotine withdrawal signs and symptoms and how to manage them.

(The history of seizure disorder makes bupropion a poor first-line cessation agent and would likely preclude its use. Considerations for use would require further risk/benefit assessment in conjunction with the patient's physician.)

3. Quit date is set for the following day with instructions to apply the first nicotine patch at bedtime the night before the quit date. The patient is instructed to perform a "clean sweep" to rid his living environment of smoking supplies, reminders, and possible triggers.

4. Social support: SJ is encouraged to communicate to his family, friends, and others regarding his current quit attempt.

5. A 2-week follow-up is set with the goal of complete abstinence and improving control of trigger situations and cravings.

References

1. Centers for Disease Control and Prevention. Annual smoking-attributable mortality, years of potential life lost, and economic costs—United States, 1995–1999. *MMWR Morb Mortal Wkly Rep.* 2002; 51:300–3.

2. NIH State-of-the-Science Conference Statement on Tobacco Use: Prevention, Cessation, and Control. NIH Consensus and State-of-the-Science Statements. Volume 23, Number 3, June 12–14, 2006.

3. Prochaska JO, DiClemente CC. Stages and processes of self-change of smoking: toward an integrative model of change. *Journal of Consulting and Clinical Psychology.* 1983; 51:390–5.

4. Velicer WF, Fava JL, Prochaska JO, et al. Distribution of smokers by stage in three representative samples. *Preventive Medicine.* 1995; 24:401–11.

5. American Psychiatric Association. *(DSM-IV-TR) Diagnostic and statistical manual of mental disorders*, 4th ed. Washington, DC: American Psychiatric Press, Inc.; 2000.

6. Heatherton TF, Kozlowski LT, Frecker RC, et al. The Fagerstrom test for nicotine dependence: a revision of the Fagerstrom tolerance questionnaire. *British Journal of Addictions.* 1991; 86:1119–27.

7. West R, McNeill A, Raw M. Smoking cessation guidelines for professionals: an update. *Thorax.* 2000; 55:989–99.

8. Vidrine JI, Cofta-Woerpl L, Daza P, et al. Smoking cessation 2: behavioral treatments. *Behavioral Medicine.* 2006; 32(3):99–109.

9. Morrell HER, Cohen LM. Cigarette smoking, anxiety and depression. *Journal of Psychopathology and Behavioral Assessment.* 2006; 28(4):283–97.

10. Cofta-Woerpl L, Wright K, Wetter D. Smoking cessation 1: pharmacological treatments. *Behavioral Medicine.* 2006; 32(2):47–56.

11. Hajek P, West R, Foulds J, et al. Randomized comparative trial of nicotine polacrilex, a transdermal patch, nasal spray, and an inhaler. *Arch Intern Med.* 1999; 159:2033–8.

12. Shiffman S, Ferguson SG, Gwaltney CJ, et al. Reduction of abstinence-induced withdrawal and craving using high-dose nicotine replacement therapy. *Psychopharmacology.* 2006; 184(3-4):637–44.

13. Holm KJ, Spencer CM. Bupropion: a review of its use in the management of smoking cessation. *Drugs.* 2000; 59:1007–24.

14. Gonazales D, Rennard SI, Nides M. Varenicline, an alpha-4, beta-2 nicotinic acetylcholine receptor partial agonist, vs sustained-release bupropion and placebo for smoking cessation: a randomized controlled trial. *JAMA.* 2006; 296:64–71.

15. Chantrix package insert. New York, NY: Pfizer Labs; September 28, 2006.

16. Okuyemi KS, Ahluwalia JS, Harris KJ. Pharmacotherapy of smoking cessation. *Arch Fam Med.* 2000; 9:270–81.

17. The Tobacco Use and Dependence Clinical Practice Guideline Panel, Staff, and Consortium Representatives. A clinical practice guideline for treating tobacco use and dependence: a U.S. public health service report. *JAMA.* 2000; 283:3244–54.

Emergency Contraception

Marianne Weber

Emergency contraception is defined as a drug or device used after unprotected intercourse or contraceptive failure to prevent pregnancy.[1] Currently, emergency contraception can be administered as a series of combination estrogen–progestin birth control or progestin-only pills or through the insertion of an intrauterine device (IUD). The progestin-only product, Plan B®, has been granted FDA approval for dispensing to women ages 18 and over without a prescription.

Data from clinical trials demonstrate higher efficacy rates with earlier versus later use of post-coital contraception.[2–4] Because pharmacists are the most accessible member of the health care team, they are in an excellent position to provide this important service directly to women in a timely manner, thereby contributing to reduced rates of unintended pregnancy.

Indications

Services can be provided for patients who request emergency contraception following unprotected intercourse or contraceptive failure within the last 120 hours,[3] and desire to not become pregnant.

Management

Development of Emergency Contraception Pill Protocols

In July 1997, five organizations in Washington state initiated a demonstration project to increase public awareness and access to emergency contraception using pharmacist collaborative agreements.[5,6] For the first time in the United States, pharmacists were able to prescribe emergency contraception pills (ECP) directly to women. Key elements of the project included educating pharmacists about ECP provision, facilitating protocol development between participating pharmacists and sponsoring prescribers, informing women about the availability of ECP, and evaluating project outcomes. Specific information regarding each component is well addressed in the references noted.

In designing a collaborative agreement allowing pharmacist provision of ECP, one should include a screening process for identifying appropriate candidates, ruling out the possibility of established ectopic or intrauterine pregnancy, and identifying additional counseling or referral needs. Discussion of sexually transmitted disease (STD) risk and routine contraception use or future pregnancy prevention are examples of potential topics to include. Acceptable regimens should be identified. Moreover, decisions should be made about whether pharmacists may prescribe them in advance as well as in response to an immediate need.

Example Procedure for Providing ECP

At our institution, we have been providing ECP for several years through an established collaborative drug therapy agreement. The procedure for this service is described here and may be adapted for implementation at another site. Each step is outlined below:

1. Obtain Emergency Contraception Screening Form for standardized charting (**Figure 9-1**).

2. Guide patient to a private area for triage process and assess the following to determine patient eligibility:

   a. *How old is she?* At our institution, patients <age 14 are referred to the pediatrics clinic or the Emergency Room for provision of ECP. Washington state law prohibits patients younger than 14 years of age from being evaluated or·treated by a pharmacist without parental consent. Note that this rule will vary according to state law. Information about adolescents' rights to consent to reproductive health, contraception, and abortion services by state can be accessed at www.guttmacher.org/sections/adolescents.php. This site is an excellent source of information and is updated monthly.

   b. *Does the patient meet inclusion criteria?* These criteria include unprotected intercourse within the last 120 hours and the desire to avoid pregnancy. Note that a woman who presents >120 hours post-coitus may be referred to the Emergency Room or her OB/GYN or primary care provider for placement of an IUD if she desires further protection. This method is effective up to 8 days after unprotected intercourse or contraceptive failure.

3. Establish the first day of the patient's last menstrual period, and whether or not other episodes of unprotected intercourse or contraceptive failure have

Patient info: Age _____   Allergies _____   PCP _____

Sexual/menstrual history: _____

	YES	NO	
1	☐	☐	Unprotected intercourse within the last 120 hours?
2			First day of your last menstrual period _____
3	☐	☐	Is this greater than 4 weeks ago?
4	☐	☐	Have you had previous unprotected sex since your last period?

If ≤120 hours postcoitus, provide ECP. If >120 hours, refer patient to the ER or Women's Clinic for placement of an IUD if she desires further protection (effective up to 8 days postcoitus).

If "YES" to questions 3 or 4, patient may already be pregnant. If at least 9 days have lapsed since last episode of unprotected intercourse, refer to _____ clinic for pregnancy screening AND dispense ECP.

5   Birth control method currently using: _____

STD education: _____

	YES	NO	
6	☐	☐	Have you had unprotected intercourse (no condom) with a new partner since your last pelvic exam?
7	☐	☐	Do you have a partner who is not monogamous?
8	☐	☐	Are you concerned that you may have been exposed to a sexually transmitted disease?

If "YES" to any of the above, dispense ECP and counsel patient regarding risk of STD transmission. Suggest she seek care for STD evaluation in _____ clinic within 1–2 weeks.

Presence of ectopic pregnancy: _____

	YES	NO	
9	☐	☐	Lower abdominal pain?
10	☐	☐	Abnormal vaginal bleeding or spotting?

If "YES" to any of the above, dispense ECP and refer patient for same-day evaluation at _____ clinic.

Plan: _____

ECP dispensed with full counseling and written instructions: (mark one)

☐   Levonorgestrel 0.75 mg, 2 tablets now, #2 (Preferred regimen)
☐   Ovral (ethinyl estradiol 50 mcg/norgestrel 0.5 mg), 2 tablets now, then 2 tablets in 12 hours, #4
☐   Promethazine 25 mg 30–60 min prior to Ovral; repeat q 6 hrs prn, #4

Instructed patient to schedule appt. in _____ clinic if no menses within 4 weeks for pregnancy test.

Pharmacist Signature_____

Figure 9-1. Emergency Contraception Screening Form

taken place since this date, because she may already be pregnant. If other episodes have occurred, provide ECP and refer patient to her primary care provider or OB/GYN for a pregnancy test.

4. Query patient about current birth control method(s) she is using and ensure she has a thorough understanding of its proper use. If she is not currently practicing any form of birth control, provide ECP and refer the patient to her primary care provider or assist her in establishing primary care in order to receive contraceptive counseling.

5. Assess presence of risk factors for STDs:
    a. Unprotected intercourse with a new partner since last pelvic exam
    b. Partner who is not monogamous

    Also inquire whether the patient is concerned that she may have been infected. If any of her answers are positive, provide ECP and recommend STD evaluation within 1 to 2 weeks with her primary care provider, OB/GYN, or local public health clinic. Remind the patient that ECP does not protect against STDs.

6. Assess presence of symptoms that may suggest an ectopic pregnancy:
    a. Lower abdominal pain
    b. Current abnormal vaginal spotting or bleeding

    If either is present, provide ECP and refer patient for same-day evaluation in her primary care or OB/GYN office, urgent care clinic, or local public health clinic.

7. Write prescription for ECP using one of the regimens noted below:
    a. *First-line therapy.* Plan B® (levonorgestrel 0.75 mg) 2 tablets as a single dose. If patient has a history of nausea with this regimen, may prescribe as 1 tablet now, with dose repeated in 12 hours. We do not routinely use the latter dosing scheme as it has been shown to be less effective than when administered as a single dose.[4]
    b. *Second-line therapy.* Ovral® (ethinyl estradiol 50 mcg/norgestrel 0.5 mg) dosed as 2 tablets now, followed by 2 tablets in 12 hours. Promethazine 25 mg tabs (#4) are also dispensed with this regimen, dosed as 1 tablet 30–60 minutes prior to Ovral; repeat q 6 hrs prn. This option should only be selected if Plan B® is unavailable because the Ovral® regimen is less effective and causes more side effects (e.g., nausea, vomiting, dizziness, fatigue) than Plan B®.[7]

8. Dispense ECP and provide full counseling. Note that as long as the patient meets inclusion criteria, no part of the protocol precludes the provision of ECP. All recommendations for additional screening, counseling, or subsequent examination are in addition to providing ECP. Routine counseling

should include discussion of the following issues appropriate to the patient's level of understanding:

a. ECP mechanism of action and expected efficacy

b. Dosing schedule

c. Potential side effects and management

d. Effect on fetus if already pregnant

e. Follow-up plan—see primary care provider or OB/GYN for pregnancy screening if no menses within 4 weeks

9. Complete documentation and send Emergency Contraception Screening Form to medical records.

Goal of Therapy

1. Prevention of unwanted pregnancy.

Clinical Pharmacy Goals

1. Provide convenient, safe, effective post-coital contraception to all women who meet criteria.

2. Educate patient regarding ECP use and encourage routine use of contraception.

3. Refer for evaluation of STDs or pregnancy when appropriate.

Outcome Measures

1. Health outcome measures: Pregnancy rates, patient satisfaction with service.

Patient and Provider Information Resources

1. Emergency Contraception Hotline: 1-888-NOT-2-LATE or http://not-2-late.com

2. http://www.path.org/publications/pub.php?id=828

3. http://www.managingcontraception.com

CASE STUDY

S: KL is a 25-year-old female who presents to your pharmacy requesting emergency contraception. She reports unprotected intercourse last night as a result of condom failure and does not wish to become pregnant. Her last menstrual period began 17 days ago, but she also had unprotected intercourse during her period without use of ECP. KL has only one partner but is unsure if he is completely faithful to her. She denies any medication allergies and symptoms of ectopic pregnancy, and is otherwise healthy.

A/P: KL meets inclusion criteria for pharmacist provision of ECP.

1. Provide Plan B® (levonorgestrel 0.75 mg) dosed as 2 tablets in a single dose, and discuss appropriate use.

2. Counsel patient regarding the following issues:

    a. *Potential pregnancy.* Since patient had unprotected intercourse roughly 2 weeks ago and has not had a period since, she may already be pregnant. Counsel that, if this is the case, Plan B® will not be effective and will not have any untoward effects on the fetus. Most urine pregnancy tests are sensitive enough to detect human chorionic gonadotropin (HCG) by 10 days gestation; therefore, refer for pregnancy screening in addition to provision of ECP. The majority of women (58%) experience their next menstrual period at the expected time or a few days early or late[7]; if she does not menstruate within the next 4 weeks, she should again be screened for pregnancy.

    b. *Condom use.* Educate patient regarding common reasons for condom failure and review proper use. Discuss efficacy of condoms compared to other contraceptive options, and encourage continued use even if she does initiate another method as she may be at risk for STDs if her partner is not monogamous.

    c. *STD risk.* Given previous and current episodes of unprotected intercourse, and lack of trust regarding her partner's sexual activity, KL may also be referred for STD evaluation within the next 1–2 weeks.

References

1. Glasier A. Emergency postcoital contraception. *NEJM.* 1997; 337:1058–64.

2. Task Force on Postovulatory Methods of Fertility Regulation. Timing of emergency contraception with levonorgestrel or the Yuzpe regimen. *Lancet.* 1999; 353:721.

3. Rodrigues I, Grou F, Joly J. Effectiveness of emergency contraceptive pills between 72 and 120 hours after unprotected intercourse. *Am J Obstet Gynecol.* 2001; 184:531–7.

4. Von Hertzen H, Piaggio G, Ding, J, et al. Low dose mifepristone and two regimens of levonorgestrel for emergency contraception: a WHO multicentre randomized trial. *Lancet.* 2002; 360:1803–10.

5. Wells ES, Hutchings J, Gardner JS, et al. Using pharmacies in Washington state to expand access to emergency contraception. *Fam Plann Perspect.* 1998 Nov–Dec; 30(6):288–90.

6. Gardner JS, Hutchings J, Fuller TS, et al. Increasing access to emergency contraception though community pharmacies: lessons from Washington state. *Fam Plann Perspect.* 2001 July–Aug; 33(4):172–5.

7. Task Force on Postovulatory Methods of Fertility Regulation. Randomised trial of levonorgestrel versus the Yuzpe regimen of combined oral contraceptives for emergency contraception. *Lancet.* 1998; 352:428–33.

Hormone Therapy and Menopause

Jennifer Kapur

Menopause is defined as the cessation of menstruation and is clinically recognized as having occurred after 12 months of amenorrhea. In the United States, the median age of menopause is 51 years (range: 41–59 years).[1] Perimenopause is the period around menopause that ends 12 months after the last menstrual period.

Indications

Hormone therapy (HT) at the lowest effective dose may be considered after the provider and patient have discussed the potential risks and benefits for the treatment of women with the following conditions:

1. Vasomotor symptoms associated with menopause:
    a. Hot flashes/flushes
    b. Night sweats
2. Vulvovaginal atrophy associated with menopause:
    a. Dryness
    b. Itching
    c. Burning
    d. Dyspareunia
    e. Atrophic vaginitis
3. Osteoporosis in women with moderate to severe menopausal symptoms: see Chapter 11 for discussion of diagnosis and treatment of osteoporosis.

Management

HT includes treatment with estrogen and combined estrogen–progestogen. The progestogen in the latter regimen is used to provide endometrial protection for women with an intact uterus.[2] HT may be given locally or systemically. Local therapy is generally recommended for patients who are using HT solely for vulvovaginal atrophy.[2] For a listing of estrogen and progestogen products available in the United States, refer to the *Postmenopausal Hormone Therapy Primer* published by the North American Menopause Society.[3]

The decision to initiate HT is not a simple one and must be individualized, weighing the benefits and risks for each woman considering treatment. Systemic HT is highly effective in relieving the vasomotor symptoms of menopause.[2,4] Systemic and local HT can treat atrophic vulvovaginal changes that may accompany menopause.[2,4] For osteoporosis, evidence shows that systemic HT can increase bone mineral density and decrease fracture risk. However, given the risks of HT and the available alternative therapies, osteoporosis should not be the sole indication for use. HT may be a suitable option for the treatment of osteoporosis in women who also have moderate to severe menopausal symptoms.[2,4]

The results of recent randomized controlled trials have led to a sharp decline in the use of HT in the prevention of chronic disease in postmenopausal women. HT has not been shown to decrease the incidence of primary or secondary coronary heart disease (CHD).[5–7] Use of HT has been associated with an increased risk of breast cancer, stroke, venous thromboembolism, cholecystitis, and endometrial cancer in women with an intact uterus taking unopposed estrogen.[1,4] Associations have also been reported between HT use and an increased risk of dementia[8] and urinary incontinence.[9] Using the lowest effective dose of HT may not only help minimize the aforementioned risks but will also help prevent or alleviate potential side effects of HT such as bloating, breast tenderness, nausea, and headaches.

Before therapy is initiated, patients must be educated about the benefits and risks of HT and complementary treatments. Lifestyle modifications (exercise, improved nutrition, limiting caffeine/alcohol/tobacco intake) and non-prescription therapies (personal lubricants, calcium supplements) are helpful to many women in reducing menopausal symptoms and/or in the prevention of osteoporosis. Patient education may also include bleeding patterns with HT and expected onset of relief in menopausal symptoms.

Goals of Therapy

1. Reduce vasomotor symptoms and/or vulvovaginal atrophy.
2. In patients with osteoporosis, increase bone mineral density and decrease fracture risk.

3. Use lowest effective dose for the shortest duration possible to decrease risks of treatment.

Clinical Pharmacy Goals

1. Identify patients non-compliant with HT and those with inappropriate regimens.

2. Ensure treatment with appropriate dosage for patient's HT indication while minimizing side effects.

3. Use a systematic approach to educate patients initiated or currently maintained on HT, documenting the education and monitoring adherence to prescribed regimens.

Outcome Measures

1. Process measures: Achieve symptom control and disease prevention in a cost-effective manner; utilize hormone replacement therapy at the lowest effective dose for the shortest duration possible based on the indication(s).

Patient Information Resources

1. http://www.menopause.org
2. http://www.nhlbi.nih.gov/health/women/index.htm
3. http://my.webmd.com/condition_center/mno

CASE STUDY

S: MR is a 52-year-old female who presents for follow-up after initiation of Prempro™ 0.625 mg/2.5 mg 1 month ago to treat vasomotor symptoms associated with menopause. She takes Prempro™ every morning upon awakening and denies any missed doses. She reports that her hot flashes and night sweats have greatly improved. She does complain of breast tenderness since starting therapy as well as nausea after she takes her daily dose. She does not have a history of breast cancer, venous thromboembolism, heart disease, or hysterectomy.

Allergies: NKDA

Current medications:

Prempro™ 0.625 mg/2.5 mg 1 tablet daily

MVI 1 tablet daily

O: BP 120/78, Weight 64 kg, Mammogram negative, Pap negative

A/P: Vasomotor symptoms associated with menopause responding well to HT; however, patient is reporting side effects of nausea and breast tenderness. *The patient has met one goal of therapy, to reduce vasomotor symptoms, but has not met the goal of using the lowest effective dose to reduce side effects. Regarding clinical pharmacy goals, she is compliant with the medication and the regimen is appropriate in that she is taking an estrogen–progestin combination because her uterus is intact.*

1. Decrease dose of Prempro™ to 0.3 mg/1.5 mg 1 tablet daily to try to alleviate nausea and breast tenderness.

2. Provide education on rationale for dose adjustment, taking Prempro™ with meals and/or at bedtime to help relieve nausea, non-pharmacologic management of hot flashes, and expected duration of therapy (i.e., use only as long as needed to relieve vasomotor symptoms).

3. Call patient in 1 month to follow up on how she is tolerating the lower dose of Prempro™ and adjust therapy as needed.

References

1. U.S. Preventive Services Task Force. Hormone therapy for the prevention of chronic conditions in postmenopausal women: recommendations for the U.S. Preventive Services Task Force. *Ann Intern Med.* 2005; 142:855–60.

2. North American Menopause Society. Recommendations for estrogen and progestogen use in peri- and postmenopausal women: October 2004 position statement of the North American Menopause Society. *Menopause.* 2004; 11:589–600.

3. North American Menopause Society. Postmenopausal Hormone Therapy Primer. Available at http://www.menopause.org/edumaterials/index.htm. Accessed June 11, 2006.

4. American College of Obstetrics and Gynecology. Executive summary. *Obstet Gynecol.* 2004; 104:S1–4.

5. Rossouw JE, Anderson GL, Prentice RL, et al. Risks and benefits of estrogen plus progestin in healthy postmenopausal women: principal results from the Women's Health Initiative randomized controlled trial. *JAMA.* 2002; 288:321–33.

6. Anderson GL, Limacher M, Assaf AR, et al. Effects of conjugated equine estrogen in postmenopausal women with hysterectomy: the Women's Health Initiative randomized controlled trial. *JAMA.* 2004; 291:1701–12.

7. Hulley S, Grady D, Bush T, et al. Randomized trial of estrogen plus progestin for secondary prevention of coronary heart disease in postmenopausal women. *JAMA.* 1998; 280:605–13.

8. Shumaker SA, Legault C, Kuller L, et al. Conjugated equine estrogens and incidence

of probable dementia and mild cognitive impairment in postmenopausal women: Women's Health Initiative Memory Study. *JAMA.* 2004; 291:2947–58.

9. Hendrix SL, Cochrane BB, Nygaard IE, et al. Effects of estrogen with and without progestin on urinary incontinence. *JAMA.* 2005; 293:935–48.

Osteoporosis

Karen Crabb

Osteoporosis, which literally means "porous bone," is a disease characterized by low bone mass and structural deterioration of bone tissue. This disease leads to increased bone fragility and risk of fracture, particularly of the hip, spine, and wrist. Osteoporosis is a major public health threat for an estimated 44 million Americans, 80% of them women.[1] In the United States, an estimated 10 million individuals have osteoporosis and an additional 34 million have low bone mass, placing them at increased risk for osteoporosis.[1] While osteoporosis is often thought of as an older person's disease, it can strike at any age.

Indications

1. Identification of patients with osteoporosis or osteopenia

   a. Diagnosis can be presumed based on the presence of risk factors and medical conditions.

   b. Definitive diagnosis from Dual Energy X-ray Absorptiometry (DEXA) scan will provide bone mineral density (BMD) T-scores to establish recommendations for treatment (Table 11-1).

Table 11-1. Bone Mineral Density

Bone Mineral Density (T-Score)	Diagnosis
>-1.0	Normal
-1.0 to -2.5	Osteopenia
<-2.5	Osteoporosis

   c. BMD of the hip is the best predictor of fractures of the hip and other
       skeletal sites.[1]
2. Identification of risk factors
   a. Modifiable risk factors include:
       • Current smoker
       • Poor calcium and vitamin D intake
       • Low physical activity
       • Greater than two alcoholic drinks per day
       • Caffeine[2]
   b. Non-modifiable risk factors include:
       • Increasing age
       • Female
       • Caucasian or Asian race
       • History of fracture in a first-degree relative
       • Dementia
       • Impaired vision
   c. Medical conditions that may be associated with an increased risk of os-
       teoporosis:
       • AIDS/HIV
       • Amyloidosis
       • Ankylosing spondylitis
       • COPD
       • Congenital porphyria
       • Cushing's syndrome
       • Eating disorders (e.g., anorexia)
       • Gastrectomy
       • Gaucher's disease
       • Hemochomatosis
       • Hemophilia
       • Hyperparathyroidism
       • Hypogonadism
       • Idiopathic scoliosis
       • Inflammatory bowel disease
       • Insulin-dependent diabetes
       • Lymphoma and leukemia
       • Malabsorption syndromes

- Mastocytosis
- Multiple sclerosis
- Pernicious anemia
- Rheumatoid arthritis
- Severe liver disease
- Spinal cord transsection
- Sprue
- Stroke/cerebrovascular accident (CVA)
- Thalassemia
- Thyrotoxicosis
- Weight loss

d. Drugs that may be associated with reduced bone mass in adults:
- Aluminum
- Anticonvulsants (phenobarbital, phenytoin)
- Cytotoxic drugs
- Glucocorticoids and adrenocorticotropin
- Gonadotropin-releasing hormone agents
- Immunosuppressants
- Lithium
- Long-term heparin use
- Progesterone (parenteral, long-acting)
- Supraphysiologic thyroxine doses
- Long-term use of total parenteral nutrition (TPN)

Management

Candidates for BMD Testing (Figure 11-1)
1. All women >65 years, regardless of risk factors
2. Women <65 years with one or more risk factors
3. Postmenopausal women who present with fractures

Treatment of Osteoporosis
1. Initiate therapy to reduce fracture risk in women with:
   a. BMD T-scores <-2.0 by hip DEXA with no risk factors
   b. BMD T-scores <-1.5 by hip DEXA with one or more risk factors
   c. Any prior vertebral or hip fractures

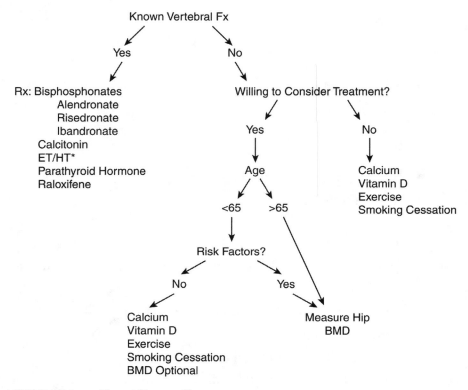

Figure 11-1. Candidates for BMD Testing

2. Counsel all patients being considered for treatment about risk factor reduction, exercise, and adequate calcium and vitamin D intake.

3. Non-pharmacologic treatment

   a. Prevent falls

      i. Remove loose wires and cords in the living area

      ii. Remove or tack down throw rugs

      iii. Ensure living area is properly illuminated, both inside and outside

      iv. Correct vision impairment or hearing deficiencies

      v. Consider hip pads for patients who have significant risk factors for falling or who have had previous hip fracture

      vi. Limit alcohol intake

      vii. Discontinue or modify pharmacotherapy that may affect balance or stability

   b. Evaluate neurologic problems

   c. Encourage smoking cessation

   d. Limit caffeine and alcohol intake

e. Encourage weight-bearing and muscle-strengthening exercises to reduce the risk of falls and fractures and increase strength and bone density

4. Pharmacologic treatment (**Table 11-2**)

a. A bisphosphonate is the first line treatment in any patient with a BMD T-Score <-2.0 and a history of falls.

b. Raloxifene or calcitonin is an option if patient is intolerant to bisphosphonates.

c. Estrogen/hormone therapy is an option for patients without risk factors for coronary artery disease (CAD), stroke, or breast cancer.

d. Calcium
    i.   All individuals should receive at least 1200 mg/day of ELEMENTAL calcium (maximum 2500 mg/day).[1]
    ii. Calcium carbonate contains 40% elemental calcium and should be taken with food for optimal absorption.[2]
    iii. Calcium citrate contains 20% elemental calcium and is recommended for patients taking proton-pump inhibitors (PPI) or H_2 blockers because acid is not required for absorption.[2]
    iv. Calcium should be taken in divided doses (maximum of 600 mg per dose) to maximize absorption.

e. Vitamin D
    i.   400 to 600 IU each day for all adults over age 50[1,2]
    ii. 800 IU/day for those at risk for deficiency (maximum 2000 IU/day)[1]

Goals of Therapy

1. Increase bone mineral density and decrease fracture risk.

2. Identify risk factors and encourage DEXA scan or further evaluation of osteoporosis.

3. Optimize therapy for prevention and treatment of osteoporosis.

Clinical Pharmacy Goals

1. Screen patients at risk for osteoporosis and facilitate appropriate evaluation.

2. Ensure appropriate pharmacologic management of patients with osteoporosis and osteopenia.

3. Educate patients regarding:
    a. Risk modification and lifestyle changes
    b. Importance of fall prevention
    c. Medication use and side effects

Table 11-2. Medications Used to Treat Osteoporosis

	Bisphosphonates	Raloxifene	Estrogen/HRT	Calcitonin	Teriparatide
Brand Names	1. Alendronate (Fosamax +/-D) 2. Ibandronate (Boniva) 3. Residronate (Actonel +/- Calcium)	Evista	Climara, Estrace, Estraderm, Estratab, Ogen, Ortho-Est, Premarin, Vivelle	Miacalcin, Calcimar, Fortical	Forteo
Product Packaging	Oral Tablets	Oral Tablets	Oral Tablets, Transdermal Patches	Nasal Spray & Injection	Injectable only
Dosing	1. 10 mg daily or 70 mg once weekly 2. 2.5 mg tab Q Day or 150 mg Q month 3. 5 mg Q Day or 35 mg once weekly	60 mg once daily	Estradiol Acetate: 0.45–1.8 mg Q Day; Conj Estrogen: 0.3–1.25 mg Q Day Esterified Estrogens: 0.75–6 mg Q Day; Estradiol: 0.25–4 mg Q Day Patch: 0.025–0.05 mg 1–2x week	1 (200 mcg) spray in 1 nostril daily	20 mcg SC daily
Reduction of Incidence of Spine Fracture*	1. 48% over 3 years 2. 50% over 3 years 3. 41–49% over 3 years	30% over 3 years	34% at the hip, 23% other fractures over 5 years	Vertebral fractures by 36%	65% after 18 months
Adverse Effects	Difficulty swallowing, gastric ulcer, esophagitis, abdominal pain, nausea, heartburn	Hot flashes, leg cramps, thromboembolic events	Thromboembolic events, increased BP, migraine, dizziness, insomnia, nausea, vomiting, abdominal cramps, diarrhea	Nasal irritation and bleeding, rhinitis, nasal sores, dryness & tenderness, back ache, arthralgia, headache	Nausea, leg cramps, dizziness, orthostatic hypotension
Special Instructions	No food x 30 minutes (60 min for Boniva); take w/water only	Separate thyroid hormone administration by 12 hours	Unopposed estrogen only for those with hysterectomy	Alternate nostrils daily	Use is limited to 18 months only; may increase digoxin toxicity
Cost	$$	$$$	$	$$	$$$$$

*Spine fracture data is obtained from the NOF's *Physician's Guide to Prevention and Treatment of Osteoporosis*.[1]

Outcome Measures

1. Process measures: Increase percentage of patients taking appropriate doses of calcium and vitamin D supplementation; increase percentage of patients diagnosed with osteoporosis receiving appropriate treatment.

2. Health outcome measures: Decrease fractures and hospital admissions among patients with identified risk factors for osteoporosis.

Patient Information Resources

1. National Osteoporosis Foundation (NOF): http://www.nof.org
2. National Institutes of Health: http://www.nih.gov
3. National Osteoporosis Society Online: http://www.nos.org.uk
4. U.S. Food and Drug Administration: http://www.fda.gov
5. The Mayo Clinic: http://www.mayoclinic.com/health/osteoporosis
6. The 2004 Surgeon General's Report on Bone Health and Osteoporosis: http://www.surgeongeneral.gov/library/bonehealth/docs/OsteoBrochure 1mar05.pdf

CASE STUDY

S: DL is a 73-year-old Caucasian woman returning to clinic 3 weeks after a minor fall causing a wrist fracture. She has no previous history of falls or fractures. She was adopted, so family history of osteoporosis is not known. DL has no history of alcohol use and quit smoking 20 years ago. Currently, DL walks for 30 minutes 3 days a week.

Allergies: NKDA

Current medications:

Calcium carbonate 500 mg/vitamin D 200 IU tid

Hydrochlorothiazide 12.5 mg daily

Multiple vitamin with iron daily

O: Height: 5 feet, 5 inches; Weight: 120 pounds

BP 122/75, HR 70

BMD T-Scores: Hip -1.9, Spine -2.1, Wrist -2.9

A: BMD measurements indicate osteopenia of the hip and spine *(BMD -1.0 to -2.5)* and osteoporosis of the wrist *(BMD <-2.5)*; however, the recent fracture indicates this patient has osteoporosis regardless of BMD measurements. *Additional risk factors include patient's age, Caucasian race, female gender, and low body weight.*

P:

1. Continue taking calcium and vitamin D tid. Continue daily multiple vitamin, which contains an additional 200 units of vitamin D. *This provides DL with 600 mg of elemental calcium and 800 units of vitamin D daily.* Encourage patient to increase dietary calcium intake to provide another 600 mg of elemental calcium *(for a total of 1200 mg elemental calcium daily).*

2. Begin alendronate 70 mg once each week. *Calcitonin nasal spray or raloxifene would be possible alternatives if the patient is not able to tolerate the side effects of a bisphosphonate. However, these agents have not demonstrated a beneficial effect for increasing bone density at the hip.*

3. Continue weight-bearing exercise 3 times a week. *There is no evidence that increasing exercise to 4 times a week has any advantage over 3 times a week.*

4. Educate patient regarding fall prevention.

5. Because DL's fall resulted in a fracture, an annual DEXA scan along with DL's annual physical may be warranted.

References

1. National Osteoporosis Foundation. Physician's Guide to Prevention and Treatment of Osteoporosis. Available at http://www.nof.org. Accessed April 2006.

2. ASHP Advantage. Preventing and Treating Osteoporosis: Therapeutic Approaches and Economic Considerations. Marybeth O'Connell, PharmD; Eugene Applebaum College of Pharmacy and Health Sciences, Wayne State University, Detroit, Michigan.

Bibliography

1. National Institutes of Health. Department of Health and Human Services. Osteoporosis: The Diagnosis. Revised November 2005. Available at http://www.nih.gov. Accessed April 2006.

2. National Institutes of Health. NIH Consensus Development Panel on Osteoporosis Prevention, Diagnosis, and Therapy; 2000. Available at http://www.nih.gov. Accessed April 2006.

3. Ettinger B, Black DM, Mitlak BH, et al, for the Multiple Outcomes of Raloxifene Evaluation (MORE) Investigators. Reduction of vertebral fracture risk in postmenopausal women with osteoporosis treated with raloxifene: results from a 3-year randomized clinical trial. *JAMA.* 1999; 282(7):637–45.

4. Cummings SR, Black DM, Thompson DE, et al. Effects of alendronate on risk of fracture in women with low bone density but without vertebral fractures: results from the fracture intervention trial. *JAMA.* 1998; 280(24):2077–82.

5. Osteoporosis: review of the evidence for prevention, diagnosis and treatment and cost-effectiveness analysis. *Osteoporosis Int.* 1998; 8(Suppl 4):S3–80.

6. Miller PD, Njeh CF, Jankowski LG, et al. What are the standards by which bone mass measurement at peripheral skeletal sites should be used in the diagnosis of osteoporosis? *J Clin Densitom.* 2002; 5(Suppl):S39–45.

7. National Osteoporosis Foundation. Health Professional's Guide to Rehabilitation of Patients with Osteoporosis; 2002.

8. Writing Group for the Women's Health Initiative Investigators. Risks and benefits of estrogen plus progestin in healthy postmenopausal women. *JAMA.* 2002; 288:321–33.

9. Delmas PD. Osteoporosis: who should be treated? *Am J Med.* 1995; 98(2A):1S–88S.

Uncomplicated Urinary Tract Infection in Women

Heidi Sawyer

Uncomplicated urinary tract infection (UTI) is a very common medical complaint for women. UTIs account for 3.6 million office visits each year in women aged 18–75 years, with 11% of women reporting at least one infection each year.[1] Uncomplicated UTIs are those infections not associated with signs or symptoms of upper urinary tract disease such as fever, chills, and flank pain. *Escherichia coli* are the causative bacteria in 75–90% of cases. *Staphylococcus saprophyticus* accounts for an additional 5–15% of cases.[1] Uncomplicated UTIs can be treated safely by a pharmacist with a minimal amount of laboratory work, as illustrated by the following protocol.

Indications

1. Patients with UTI are defined as having both of the following:
   a. Women, ages 18–55 years old with symptoms of dysuria, urgency, frequency, or hematuria. Patients must have one or more of these symptoms.
   b. Urine dip positive for leukocyte esterase and/or nitrite.

Exclusion Criteria[2]

Patients meeting any of the following exclusion criteria would not be eligible for the uncomplicated UTI protocol:

1. Urine dip negative
2. Fever $\geq 100.5°F$ or $38°C$
3. Nausea, vomiting, or abdominal pain

4. Diabetes

5. Pregnancy

6. Immunosuppression (e.g., cancer, HIV+)

7. Symptoms >7 days

8. Symptoms of vaginitis (itching or discharge)

9. Recent urinary stones

10. Renal or urologic abnormalities other than stress incontinence

11. Gross hematuria in women >50 years

12. Treatment for UTI within the last 2 weeks

13. Catheterization or other urologic procedure within the last 2 weeks

14. Discharge from hospital or nursing home within the last 2 weeks

Management

Figure 12-1 provides a flow chart of the steps involved. First, obtain a medication allergy history for the following situations.

1. For patients with less than two UTIs in the last year:

    a. If local *E. coli* resistance <20% and no allergy to sulfa, treat with trimethoprim/sulfamethoxazole 1 DS tablet bid for 3 days unless risk factors for resistance are present (see below).[1,3]

    b. Risk factors associated with antibiotic resistance to trimethoprim/sulfamethoxazole:[4]

        i.   Antibiotic treatment, especially with trimethoprim/sulfamethoxazole, within the last 3 months

        ii. Current use of antibiotics

        iii. Hospitalization within the last 3 months[5]

        iv. Diabetes mellitus

    c. If local *E. coli* resistance ≥20%, sulfa allergy, or risk factors for resistance to trimethoprim/sulfamethoxazole, treat with:[1,3]

        i.   Nitrofurantoin SR 100 mg po bid x 7 days or 50 mg qid x 7 days

        ii. Ciprofloxacin 250 mg po bid x 3 days. Use as second-line agent to prevent antibiotic resistance to quinolones.[2]

    d. Consider addition of phenazopyridine 100 mg po tid x 2 days to reduce patient discomfort.[1]

2. For patients with two or more UTIs in the last year:

    a. Obtain urinalysis (UA) and culture prior to dispensing medication.

    b. Schedule (or recommend, depending on practice setting) follow-up with primary care provider (PCP).

Carefully selected patients with symptoms of dysuria or urgency may be safely managed without a visit with the physician or health care specialist (HCS). These guidelines apply only to patients who do not have an exclusion as noted in the guidelines. Eligible patients will be triaged, treated, and counseled according to these guidelines by a pharmacist or a nurse.

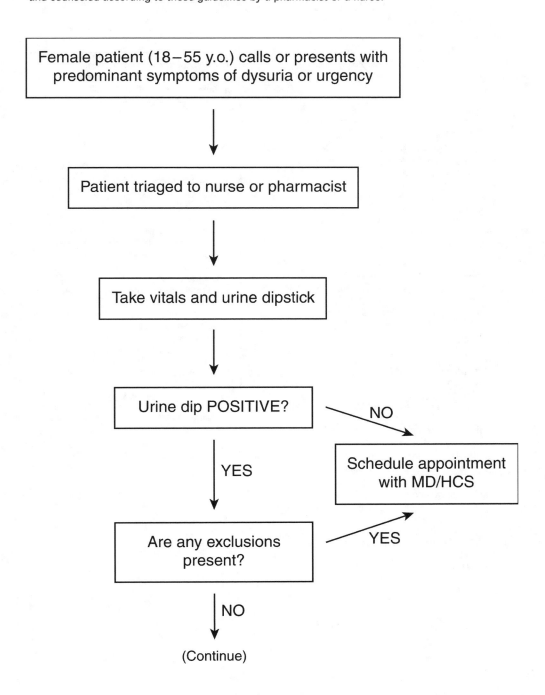

Figure 12-1. Acute Uncomplicated UTI Protocol (continued on next page)

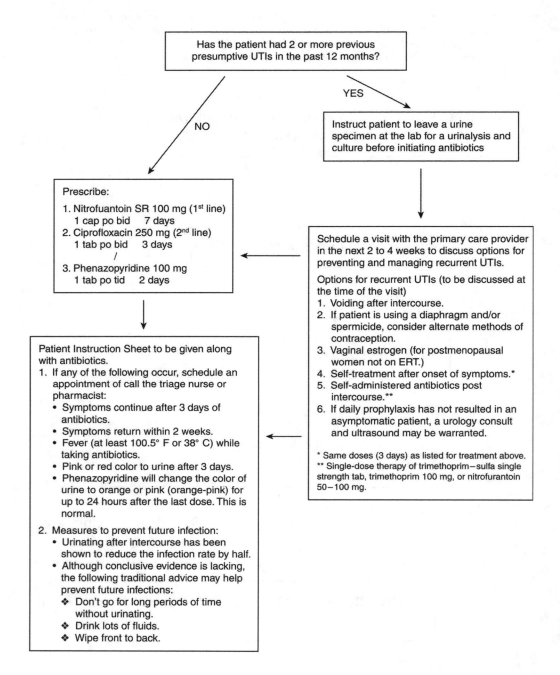

Has the patient had 2 or more previous presumptive UTIs in the past 12 months?

NO

YES

Instruct patient to leave a urine specimen at the lab for a urinalysis and culture before initiating antibiotics

Prescribe:

1. Nitrofuantoin SR 100 mg (1st line)
   1 cap po bid   7 days
2. Ciprofloxacin 250 mg (2nd line)
   1 tab po bid   3 days
   /
3. Phenazopyridine 100 mg
   1 tab po tid   2 days

Schedule a visit with the primary care provider in the next 2 to 4 weeks to discuss options for preventing and managing recurrent UTIs.

Options for recurrent UTIs (to be discussed at the time of the visit)
1. Voiding after intercourse.
2. If patient is using a diaphragm and/or spermicide, consider alternate methods of contraception.
3. Vaginal estrogen (for postmenopausal women not on ERT.)
4. Self-treatment after onset of symptoms.*
5. Self-administered antibiotics post intercourse.**
6. If daily prophylaxis has not resulted in an asymptomatic patient, a urology consult and ultrasound may be warranted.

* Same doses (3 days) as listed for treatment above.
** Single-dose therapy of trimethoprim–sulfa single strength tab, trimethoprim 100 mg, or nitrofurantoin 50–100 mg.

Patient Instruction Sheet to be given along with antibiotics.
1. If any of the following occur, schedule an appointment of call the triage nurse or pharmacist:
   • Symptoms continue after 3 days of antibiotics.
   • Symptoms return within 2 weeks.
   • Fever (at least 100.5° F or 38° C) while taking antibiotics.
   • Pink or red color to urine after 3 days.
   • Phenazopyridine will change the color of urine to orange or pink (orange-pink) for up to 24 hours after the last dose. This is normal.

2. Measures to prevent future infection:
   • Urinating after intercourse has been shown to reduce the infection rate by half.
   • Although conclusive evidence is lacking, the following traditional advice may help prevent future infections:
     ❖ Don't go for long periods of time without urinating.
     ❖ Drink lots of fluids.
     ❖ Wipe front to back.

Figure 12-1. Acute Uncomplicated UTI Protocol (continued)

    c. Discuss preventative measures:

       i. Urination after intercourse

      ii. Although conclusive evidence is lacking, the patient may help to prevent infections by avoiding long time periods between urination, drinking lots of fluids, and wiping front to back.

    d. Prescribe treatment for UTI as outlined under #2 above.

3. Instruct all patients to return for care for any of the following:

    a. Symptoms continue after 3 days of antibiotics

    b. Symptoms return within 2 weeks

    c. Fever (at least 100.5° F or 38° C) while taking antibiotics

    d. Pink or red color to urine after 3 days. Remember, phenazopyridine will change the color of urine to orange or pink for up to 24 hours after the last dose. This is normal.

Goals of Therapy

1. Appropriate treatment of uncomplicated UTIs.

2. Prevention of clinical failure, defined as a phone call or additional visit within 2 weeks for a UTI-related symptom.[6]

Clinical Pharmacy Goals

1. Ensure treatment with effective antibiotic based on local resistance rates for *E. coli.*

2. Educate patients regarding preventative measures and when to seek further care.

Outcome Measures

1. Process measures: Appropriately treat uncomplicated UTIs in a cost-effective manner in order to prevent return visits, repeat courses of antibiotics, and antibiotic resistance; increase patient awareness of methods to prevent UTIs.

Patient Information Resources

1. Web MD: http://www.webmd.com/hw/infection/hw57228.asp

2. National Kidney and Urologic Disease Information Clearinghouse: http://kidney.niddk.nih.gov/kudiseases/pubs/utiadult/

3. National Women's Health Information Center: http://womenshealth.gov/faq/Easyread/uti-etr.htm

CASE STUDY

S: RM is a 24-year-old female who presents to a clinic in Seattle, Washington, with symptoms of urinary urgency, frequency, and pain with urination. RM reports that symptoms began 3 days ago. Her urine dip is positive for leukocyte esterase and nitrites. She is referred to the pharmacist.

On further questioning, RM reports feeling well, aside from the symptoms listed above. She denies any fever, abdominal pain, nausea, vomiting, vaginal discharge, vaginal itching, or possible pregnancy. She denies any other medical conditions such as diabetes or any condition causing immunosuppression. She denies any treatment for UTI in the last 2 weeks as well as any urologic abnormalities or hospitalizations. She reports last treatment for UTI 18 months ago and does note treatment with amoxicillin 2 months ago for an unrelated infection.

Allergies: NKDA

Current medications: Levothyroxine 100 mcg daily

O: Vital signs: BP 112/70, HR 76, T 36° C

A/P: Uncomplicated UTI per urine dip without the presence of any exclusion criteria.

1.   Prescribe nitrofurantoin SR 100 mg, 1 cap po bid x 7 days. *Patient has presented for care in a region of the country with trimethoprim–sulfamethoxazole resistance >20%. Therefore, treatment with trimethoprim–sulfamethoxazole is not recommended. Ciprofloxacin is considered a second-line agent in an attempt to prevent quinolone resistance.*

2.   Prescribe phenazopyridine 100 mg 1 tab po tid x 2 days and educate patient about side effects of this medication. *Would discuss orange-to-pink discoloration of urine, which can persist for 24 hours after the last dose of phenazopyridine.*

3.   Provide patient education about when to seek additional care and how to prevent UTIs in the future. Instruct patient to contact the clinic if symptoms persist after 3 days of antibiotic treatment; symptoms return within 2 weeks of starting antibiotics; fever appears while taking antibiotics; or pink or red color to urine occurs 24 hours after completing phenazopyridine. Patient can attempt to prevent UTIs by avoiding long periods between urinating, drinking lots of fluid, and wiping front to back.

References

1. Fihn SD. Acute uncomplicated urinary tract infection in women. *N Engl J Med.* 2003; 349(3):259–66.

2. Personal Communication: UW Department of OB/GYN, April 20, 2006. Eckert L.

3. Karlowsky JA, Thornsberry C, Jones ME, et al. Susceptibility of antimicrobial-resistant urinary *Escherichia coli* isolates to fluoroquinolones and nitrofurantoin. *Clin Infect Dis.* 2003; 36:183–7.

4. Hooton TM, Besser R, Foxman B, et al. Acute uncomplicated cystitis in an era of increasing antibiotic resistance: a proposed approach to empirical therapy. *Clin Infect Dis.* 2004; 39:75–80.

5. Wright SW, Wrenn KD, Hayes MI. Trimethoprim-sulfamethoxazole resistance among urinary coliform isolates. *J Gen Intern Med.* 1999; 14:606–9.

6. Brown PD, Freeman A, Foxman B. Prevalence and predictors of trimethoprim-sulfamethoxazole resistance among uropathogenic *Escherichia coli* isolates in Michigan. *Clin Infect Dis.* 2002; 34:1061–6.

Treatment Guidelines for Human Immunodeficiency Virus-1 Infected Adults

Beth Hykes

To date, approximately 65 million people have been infected with the human immunodeficiency virus-1 (HIV) and more than 25 million people have died from acquired immunodeficiency syndrome (AIDS) since it was first recognized in 1981.[1] Despite global efforts at prevention, there are more new HIV infections every year than AIDS-related deaths. Guidelines have been established and routinely updated to assist health care providers in the management of HIV-infected individuals. Pharmacists have a unique opportunity to impact patient care not only with their drug therapy knowledge, but also by providing a link between health care providers and patients.

Indications

Antiretroviral Therapy for the Chronically Infected HIV Patient (National Guidelines)[2]

Established infection: positive ELISA test confirmed by Western Blot

(See **Table 13-1** for indications on initiating therapy based on CD4 cell count and viral load.)

Highly Active Antiretroviral Therapy (HAART) Protocol (Institutional Guidelines: Harborview Medical Center, Seattle, Washington)[3]

Please refer to **Appendix 13-1**. Patient meets national guidelines above and the following:

1. Patient is naïve to HAART *or*
2. Patient has been off HAART for >6 months

Table 13-1. Indications for Initiating Antiretroviral Therapy in the Chronically Infected HIV-1 Adult[2]

Clinical Category	CD4 T Cell Count	Plasma HIV Viral Load	Recommendation
Symptomatic (AIDS, severe symptoms)	Any value	Any value	Treat
Asymptomatic, AIDS	<200 cells/mm^3	Any value	Treat
Asymptomatic	>200 cells/mm^3 but <350 cells/mm^3	Any value	Treatment should be offered, with consideration of pros and cons
Asymptomatic	>350 cells/mm^3	<100,000 copies/mL	Most clinicians would defer therapy
Asymptomatic	>350 cells/mm^3	>100,000 copies/mL	Defer therapy

Management[2]

1. Recommended combination therapy for the management of HIV-1 infected treatment-naïve individuals (**Table 13-2**)

2. Factors to consider when selecting an initial regimen[2]

   a. *Results of genotype resistance testing.* Resistance assays are recommended in the following areas of clinical practice:

      i. Determining initial antiretroviral therapy in both acute and chronic infection (to detect if resistant virus was transmitted and to guide treatment decisions)

      ii. In the case of virologic failure (to assist in selecting active drugs for a new regimen)

      iii. In pregnant patients (to guide treatment decisions)

   b. *Adherence potential.* Prior to initiating HAART, clinicians must assess the patient's readiness to take medication. The patient's report of adherence to current or previous medications should be reviewed to determine if there is a history of non-adherence. Any potential barriers must be addressed prior to initiating therapy. Examples of strategies to improve or maximize adherence include providing education on medication dosing; simplifying regimens; informing the patient of specific food/water requirements; anticipating and treating adverse drug effects using a team approach with pharmacists, nutritionists, and counselors; and utilizing reminder aids such as pill boxes.

Table 13-2. Recommended Combination Therapy for the Management of HIV-1 Infected Treatment-Naïve Individuals[2]

Type of Regimen*	Description*	Note*
NNRTI based	1 NNRTI + 2 NRTI	Preferred and alternative options exist based on efficacy and tolerability. See guidelines[2] for most recently recommended agents.
PI based	1 PI + 2 NRTI	
NRTI based	3 NRTI	To be used only when a preferred or alternative NNRTI or PI-based regimen cannot or should not be used as first-line therapy.

*NRTI = nucleoside reverse transcriptase inhibitor; NNRTI = non-nucleoside reverse transcriptase inhibitor; PI = protease inhibitor.

c. *Medication allergies.* The following antiretroviral agents are sulfonamide derivatives and must be used with caution in patients with a known sulfonamide allergy:

  i. Amprenavir

  ii. Darunavir

  iii. Fos-amprenavir

  iv. Tipranavir

  Other sulfonamides used in the management of opportunistic infections include:

  i. Dapsone

  ii. Trimethoprim–sulfamethoxazole

  iii. Sulfadiazine

d. *Potential adverse drug effects.* Adverse drug effects have been reported with all antiretroviral agents and are among the most common reasons for medication non-adherence and for switching or discontinuing therapy. When selecting a regimen that a patient will be taking long term, health care personnel must consider a patient's lifestyle and any history of drug intolerance. Pharmacists play a critical role in educating patients about potential adverse drug effects before they occur. Providing patients with clear instructions on how to identify and manage adverse effects enables them to take an active role in their care.

e. *Baseline CD4 cell count.* Pre-treatment CD4 cell count must be considered because it may impact the choice of antiretroviral therapy. For example, symptomatic, sometimes serious, and even fatal hepatic events (accompanied by rash in approximately 50% of cases) occur with significantly higher frequency in female patients with pre-nevirapine CD4 T cell counts >250 cells/mm³ or in male patients with pre-nevirapine CD4 T cell counts >400 cells/mm³. Nevirapine should not be initiated in these patients unless the benefit clearly outweighs the risk.

f. *Gender.* Females are at higher risk of certain antiretroviral adverse effects, including:

   i.   Hepatic events and Stevens-Johnson syndrome/toxic epidermal necrosis from nevirapine

   ii. Rash from nevirapine or tipranavir

   iii. Lactic acidosis/hepatic steatosis with or without pancreatitis from nucleoside analogues

g. *Potential drug–drug interactions.* A thorough review of a patient's current list of medications must be completed prior to starting an antiretroviral regimen to avoid potential drug–drug interactions. Current medications should include prescription and over-the-counter preparations, illicit substances, and naturopathic remedies. A review should be conducted whenever a new medication is added or removed from a patient's list of active medications to avoid an adverse drug interaction.

h. *Convenience.* Consider the most convenient regimen (e.g., low pill burden, simple dosing, limited food/fluid restriction). Once-daily dosing options exist in all antiretroviral classes except for fusion inhibitors. Protease inhibitor (PI) pill burden has been dramatically reduced with the use of ritonavir boosting. Each regimen has its own limitations and advantages and must be taken into consideration to meet a particular patient's desires. For example, the PI lopinavir/ritonavir may be dosed once daily or twice daily in a treatment-naïve patient. However, the once-daily dosing option is associated with a higher incidence of gastrointestinal intolerance and achieves a lower trough concentration than the twice-daily dosing.

i. *Co-morbidity or concomitant conditions.* Existing co-morbidities such as tuberculosis, liver disease, depression or mental illness, cardiovascular disease, and chemical dependency may impact choice of regimen for a particular patient. For example, efavirenz may cause several nervous system side effects, including depression and exacerbation of psychiatric disorders or hallucinations. Risk factors for these adverse effects include pre-existing or unstable psychiatric illnesses. Patients at risk for cardiovascular disease may benefit from a regimen with a PI that has less of an effect on lipid profile, such as atazanavir.

j. *Pregnancy potential.* Selection of antiretroviral combinations should take into account known safety, efficacy, and pharmacokinetic data of each agent during pregnancy. Current Public Health Service guidelines should be consulted when designing a regimen for a pregnant patient. For pregnant women, an additional goal of therapy is prevention of mother-to-child transmission, with a goal of viral suppression to <1,000 copies/mL to reduce the risk of transmission to the fetus and newborn. Pregnant women are at higher risk of developing hepatic events from nevirapine and lactic acidosis/hepatic steatosis with or without pancreatitis from nucleoside analogues (especially with the nucleoside backbone of stavudine + didanosine). Efavirenz is not recommended in the first trimester of pregnancy or in sexually active women with child-bearing potential who are not using effective contraception.

3. Referral of a patient to the HAART protocol[3]

   The HAART protocol was developed in 1998 by our institution in order to address the problem of patient adherence (according to pharmacy refill records). The protocol uses a multidisciplinary approach to patient care, involving the patient's provider, a pharmacist, a nutritionist, and a case manager who work closely together as a team. This multidisciplinary approach to patient care is designed to improve long-term success with HAART.

   The protocol is initiated by the patient's provider. The suggested treatment regimen and any potential barriers to adherence are documented in a routing form (see Appendix 13-1, **Figure 13A-1**), which is reviewed by all participating disciplines. Potential barriers to success with HAART include financial obstacles, fear of side effects, potential drug interactions, and conflict between the regimen and a patient's lifestyle. Each discipline approaches issues that they can address and proposes a solution after a visit with the patient. Each discipline makes a recommendation to either initiate or postpone HAART based on its assessment. Overall, the HAART protocol is intended to assess a patient's readiness and willingness to begin antiretroviral therapy. At this time, patients also receive education about HAART (specifically about the medications in the patient's proposed regimen), emphasizing the importance of adherence for therapeutic success and the prevention of resistance development.

4. Factors to consider when changing therapy due to treatment failure:[2]

   a. *Adherence.* Assess the patient's adherence to the regimen. For incomplete adherence, if possible, identify and address the underlying causes for non-adherence (e.g., access to medication, active substance abuse, loss of insurance, forgetfulness) and simplify the regimen by decreasing pill burden or dosing frequency.

   b. *Medication intolerance.* Assess any adverse drug effects the patient may be experiencing. Address and review the likely duration of side effects (e.g., limited duration of gastrointestinal side effects of some regimens).

Management strategies for intolerance may include:

i.   Use symptomatic treatment

ii. Use another drug within the same class (e.g., change to lopinavir/ ritonavir for atazanavir-related jaundice)

iii. Change drug class [e.g., from a non-nucleotide reverse transcriptase inhibitor (NNRTI) to a PI, or vice versa if necessary]

c. *Pharmacokinetic issues*

i.   Review food/fasting requirements for each medication

ii. Review recent history of gastrointestinal symptoms to assess the likelihood of short-term malabsorption

iii. Review concomitant medications and dietary supplements for possible adverse drug–drug interactions and make appropriate substitutions for antiretroviral agents and/or concomitant medications, if possible

d. *Suspected drug resistance.* Obtain resistance testing while the patient is taking the failing regimen or within 4 weeks after regimen discontinuation. Drug resistance testing is not recommended for persons with a viral load <1,000 copies/mL because amplification of the virus is unreliable. Treatment options for a failing regimen must be considered on a case-by-case basis. Please refer to the national guidelines for support with this complex situation.[2]

5. Prevention and management of opportunistic infections[4]

Despite the advances in antiretroviral therapy over the past 10 years, patients continue to be at risk for opportunistic infections. With the initiation of HAART and immune reconstitution, prophylactic therapy for opportunistic infections is no longer a lifelong commitment. Pharmacists can help screen patients to ensure appropriate initiation and discontinuation of prophylactic and treatment regimens of opportunistic infections. (A complete discussion of opportunistic infections is beyond the scope of the chapter.)

Goals of Therapy

1. Increase in CD4 T cell count by 100–150 cells/ mm^3/year, with an accelerated response in the first 3 months. Subsequent increases with good virologic control show an average increase of 100 cells/mm^3/year for the subsequent few years until a plateau is reached.

2. Viral load or HIV RNA below the limits of detection: <50 copies/mL for the HIV reverse transcriptase polymerase chain reaction assay.

Clinical Pharmacy Goals

1. The pharmacist's role in the HAART protocol:

   a. Assess a patient's knowledge of HIV and the medications used for its treatment.

      i. Educate patients on potential adverse effects and their management strategies for HAART. Two examples follow:

         • Lopinavir/ritonavir commonly causes diarrhea. Consider providing patients with a prescription for loperamide in the event that it becomes necessary. In addition to the pharmacist, the patient speaks with a nutritionist to learn about foods that may help to alleviate diarrhea, such as rice or applesauce.

         • Up to 50% of patients taking efavirenz experience adverse central nervous system effects, including sedation, dizziness, confusion, and abnormal thinking. Patients are instructed to take their medication in the evening just before bedtime to avoid the negative adverse effects. They are also educated that these adverse effects generally subside within 2–3 weeks.

      ii. Review patient's current therapy to avoid potential drug–drug interactions.

      iii. Identify the need for dose adjustments based on impaired renal or hepatic function and for low body weight. For example, all nucleoside reverse transcriptase inhibitors (NRTIs), with the exception of abacavir, require renal dose adjustment in patients with renal insufficiency.

   b. Provide information that will better enable the patient to take his or her medications appropriately and achieve better clinical outcomes.

      i. Educate patients about the need for medication-related dietary requirements. Two examples follow:

         • Certain PIs require food for absorption such as atazanavir, darunavir, nelfinavir, ritonavir, saquinavir, and tipranavir.

         • Certain antiretroviral agents require that they be taken on an empty stomach (1 hour before or 2 hours after a meal) such as efavirenz, didanosine EC, and indinavir (when used as a PI, although using indinavir as a sole PI is not recommended).

      ii. Provide strategies to handle late or missed doses:

         • Patients should never double up on doses if they miss a dose. Rather, they should take the dose as soon as they remember it. If it is closer to the time that the next dose is due, they should omit the missed dose and take the next dose at the scheduled time.

- A general rule of thumb is that if a dosing interval is 12 hours apart, patients should take a late dose within 6 hours of the time it was due. If it is after 6 hours, they should wait until the next dose is due and resume their normal dosing schedule.

c. Identify potential barriers to medication adherence and offer interventions to reduce those barriers.

    i. Educate patients regarding the importance of adherence.

    ii. Provide the patient with methods to increase adherence such as the use of medication boxes, daily reminders with alarm devices, association with daily activities, and patient support groups.

d. Review key points

This should be done both prior to the initial dispensation of the medications and at the 2-week refill to assess the development of side effects or other problems that could result in medication non-adherence or discontinuation of therapy.

Outcome Measures

1. Process measures: Restore and preserve immunologic function; maximally and durably suppress viral load.

2. Health outcome measures: Reduce HIV-related morbidity and mortality; improve quality of life.

Patient Information Resources

1. The complete HIV/AIDS resource: http://www.thebody.com

2. Information on HIV and AIDS: http://www.aidsmap.com

3. Information for people living with HIV/AIDS: http://www.projectinform.org

CASE STUDY

S: A 30-year-old HIV-infected woman presents to an HIV Clinic for routine follow-up. She has no HIV-related symptoms and has had no AIDS-defining illnesses. Her only complaint today is increasing fatigue, which she has attributed to her new waitress position. She is so busy that she does not have time to eat a meal during her shift. She is concerned that her employer will learn of her diagnosis if she is unable to perform her job. She often misses doses of her antidepressant because she fears that her co-workers will see her taking her medication and be curious about her diagnosis. She occasionally takes a medication for heartburn when she is uncomfortable at work. She has never required antiretroviral therapy. She presents today to review her recent laboratory blood work taken 1 week ago. After her appointment, the physician recommends initiating atazanavir 300 mg daily, ritonavir 100 mg daily + Truvada® (emtricitabine 200 mg/tenofovir 300 mg) 1 tablet daily.

Allergies: Augmentin® = rash, no known environmental allergies or food allergies

Current medications:

Ranitidine 150 mg twice a day

Citalopram 20 mg daily

O: Recent laboratory tests:

1 week ago

CD4 cell count: 330 cells/mm^3

HIV RNA level: 175,000 copies/mL

SCr: 0.9 mg/dL

AST/ALT: 38/54

3 months prior

CD4 cell count: 370 cells/mm^3

HIV RNA level: 65,000 copies/mL

SCr: 0.8 mg/dL

AST/ALT: 39/49

A/P:

1. The patient meets criteria for starting antiretroviral therapy according to the national guidelines based on her most recent CD4 cell count. Therapy should be offered after consideration of the pros and cons of therapy. *Potential benefits of deferred therapy include avoidance of treatment-related negative effects on quality of life and drug-related toxicities. Deferred therapy would also allow more time for the patient to have a greater understanding of treatment demands. Potential risks of deferred therapy include the possibility that damage to the immune system, which might otherwise be salvaged by earlier therapy, is irreversible.*

2. The patient should be referred to the institution-specific antiretroviral initiation therapy protocol before starting her regimen as she meets the national guidelines and is naïve to therapy. *Institutional guidelines usually require that assessments by social work and nutrition be completed in addition to the pharmacist assessment before an individual begins antiretroviral therapy.*

a. Potential barriers to adherence should be discussed. *Her history of non-adherence to her current antidepressant therapy needs to be addressed before she begins HAART. Ensure that the patient understands the importance of adherence and that she is ready to commit to taking therapy before recommending that she start HAART.* Provide patient with education about how non-adherence leads to drug resistance, may limit future treatment options, and ultimately leads to therapeutic failure. *A few suggestions to assist the patient with adherence include:*

   i. *Ask the patient to monitor her adherence to her antidepressant therapy to ensure that she is no longer missing doses prior to starting HAART. This may be a helpful indicator that she may be able to take her HAART regimen consistently.*

   ii. *Suggest ways to ensure that she takes her doses in a private place (at home or in a personal area at work) so that she does not miss doses in the future.*

   iii. *Ensure that the patient has regular follow-up for her depression so that her condition is managed and does not limit her ability to adhere to her regimen.*

   iv. *Identify whether treatment-related adverse effects will limit her from adhering to her regimen. For example, a regimen that causes significant diarrhea would limit her ability to function as a waitress.*

b. The patient's history of medication allergies will not interfere with the proposed regimen.

c. In an effort to design a regimen that the patient can adhere to for the long term, provide education about the proposed antiretroviral regimen including potential short- and long-term side effects, dosing convenience, and pill burden. *This information will enable the patient to take an active role in fitting the regimen into her lifestyle. It will also prepare her for what to expect from her regimen before she begins therapy. Providing this information to the patient before she begins therapy will identify if there are any potential barriers to success with the regimen itself. For example, is the patient uncomfortable with the number of pills in the regimen or so fearful of the potential adverse effects that it may prevent her from being adherent to the regimen?*

   i. *The short-term side effects of the proposed regimen may include diarrhea (mild), nausea, abdominal discomfort (ritonavir and atazanavir), and increased bilirubin (atazanavir). The patient should report any jaundice and must* get blood work done for evaluation. The patient should contact her physician or pharmacy if any gastrointestinal side effects are bothersome. Other side effects may include nausea, upset stomach, headaches, and fatigue (Truvada®).

   ii. The long-term side effects of the regimen may include hepatotoxiticy, insulin resistance/diabetes mellitus, fat maldistribution, and osteonecrosis (PIs). Truvada® may cause lactic acidosis with hepatic steatosis with long-term use.

   iii. The patient will be able to take all three medications together once a day with a snack when it is convenient with her work schedule.

d. Take into consideration pre-treatment CD4 cell count and gender because these factors may affect choice of antiretroviral therapy. The patient's pre-treatment CD4 cell count is 330 cells/mm³. When considering treatment options, the drug nevirapine should be avoided since there is a greater risk of hepatotoxicity in female patients with high CD4 cell counts (>250 cells/mm³).

e. Consider current medication therapy and potential drug–drug interactions (including over-the-counter medication, natural medicine, or illicit substances). She intermittently takes a medication for heartburn. Many antiretroviral medications cannot be taken with acid-suppressing agents or may require that they be taken at different times than antacid administration.

   i. Instruct the patient that she will be able to continue taking her H-2 blocker; however, she must take it 12 hours apart from the time that she takes her antiretroviral regimen.

   ii. Many antidepressants can be taken safely with HAART; however, the levels of the antidepressants may be elevated due to an interaction with PIs. A general recommendation is to use lower doses of antidepressants and to slowly increase the dose when used in combination with HAART. The patient reports that she takes citalopram 20 mg daily. Levels of citalopram may be elevated; however, no dose adjustment is necessary since citalopram has many paths of metabolism. Patient is unlikely to experience any side effects with the addition of her HAART regimen. Instruct patient to call if she experiences any new adverse effects with the start of her regimen, including nausea, sweating, insomnia, drowsiness, and dry mouth, which may indicate that her citalopram levels are elevated.

f. Consider current dietary habits. Certain antiretroviral regimens require food for absorption or are recommended to be taken *with food to minimize side effects. Other regimens must be taken on an empty stomach or with plenty of water.* Atazanavir with ritonavir must be taken with a snack or small meal to ensure adequate absorption. Assist patient with ideas of what she can eat as a snack when she takes her medication once daily.

g. Consider co-morbidities (e.g., is her depression under control and/or might it impact her ability to adhere to the regimen) and pregnancy potential.

   i. Ensure that her depression has been evaluated and managed so that it does not have a negative impact on adherence. *Certain antiretroviral medications should not be used in a patient with a history of depression that is not well managed. For example, efavirenz may exacerbate depression in a patient with a pre-existing history.*

   ii. Consider potential for pregnancy and how this may impact choice of therapy. *This patient is of child-bearing age. Efavirenz is a known teratogen and should be avoided in women of child-bearing age who are at risk of becoming pregnant and not using an effective means of birth control.*

h. Review factors that may affect antiretroviral dosing such as baseline renal and hepatic function and weight. *The patient's renal and hepatic functions are within normal limits and, therefore, her antiretroviral medications do not require dose adjustments at this time.*

i. Educate patient about the need for ongoing laboratory evaluation to monitor therapy and to prevent toxicity.

j. Follow-up with patient for a second visit prior to starting HAART to review teaching points once a regimen has been decided.

k. Follow-up with patient 2 weeks after starting HAART to determine if patient is adhering to and tolerating the regimen and if any new questions have arisen.

References

1. UNAIDS. Report on the Global AIDS Epidemic, 2006. Available at: www.unaids.org. Accessed September 25, 2006.

2. Department of Health and Human Services. Guidelines for the Use of Antiretroviral Agents in HIV-1 Infected Adults and Adolescents. Oct 10, 2006. Available at http://AIDSinfo.nih.gov. Accessed October 18, 2006.

3. Madison Clinic HAART Protocol, Established February 1998, Seattle Washington Harborview Medical Center.

4. Treating Opportunistic Infections Among HIV-Infected Adults and Adolescents. December 17, 2004. Available at http://AIDSinfo.nih.gov. Accessed April 13, 2006.

Appendix 13-1: Highly Active Antiretroviral Therapy (HAART) Protocol

Why Do We Have the HAART Protocol?

The combination antiretrovirals have demonstrated success with regards to reductions in morbidity, mortality, and overall health care costs for HIV+ persons.[1-3] As adherence decreases, viral loads and the risk of progression to AIDS increase linearly, however.[4-6] Non-adherence among persons with chronic illnesses is widespread; among those taking HAART (Highly Active Antiretroviral Therapy), 40–60% are less than 90% adherent.[7-11] The level of adherence required for success, however, is thought to be a staggering 95% or greater.[8] During 1997, a brief look at pharmacy refill histories identified an adherence problem among our patients. To address this problem, a multidisciplinary HAART Adherence Committee was established, and the HAART Protocol was implemented as clinic policy in February 1998.

The Protocol has been designed to ensure that all patients receive education about HAART and the importance of adherence for therapeutic success and prevention of resistance development. In addition, the patient's readiness to begin antiretrovirals is assessed as well as identification and elimination of potential barriers to adherence prior to initiation of HAART.

The following is a summary of the differences between the "**Pre-HAART**" Protocol and the "**On-HAART**" Protocol. It should also be noted that the Pre-HAART Protocol is *required* to begin antiretrovirals at Madison Clinic, and the On-HAART Protocol is *highly suggested* but not required for those patients identified.

1. Patients required to be enrolled in **Pre-HAART** Protocol before starting HAART

    a. Patients naïve to HAART therapy (may have received nucleosides in the past)

    b. Patients who have been off HAART for >6 months

2. Patients eligible to be enrolled in **On-HAART** Protocol

    a. Patients on HAART considering a change due to intolerance or virologic failure

    b. Patients on HAART who have been identified as having adherence problems

    c. Patients already started on HAART (from other providers or primary infection clinic) who desire education about the regimen

    d. Patients off HAART for <6 months who are considering restarting therapy

e. Any patient not meeting the above criteria who wishes to learn more about antiretrovirals through interdisciplinary education

We ask that patients not be routed through the HAART Protocol on their first visit to the clinic. This is simply overwhelming to the patient and is rarely appropriate. Exceptions to this rule are patients from out of town who are here only for HAART therapy and pregnant women. We do ask that such patients be sent through the Protocol as soon as possible so that they will benefit from the counseling early in therapy.

Who Is *Not* Required to Go Through the HAART Protocol?

Patients with the following conditions are not required to go through the HAART Protocol, as HAART is the only available treatment:

* Pregnancy
* Dementia/PML
* Severe ITP

If patients have one of the conditions listed above, they will receive medications on the day of the appointment and basic drug information from pharmacy. Nursing will schedule their appointments with each discipline to take place in the following weeks.

What Factors Have Been Associated with Non-Adherence?

* Mental health (especially depression and anxiety)
* Substance use
* Negative attitudes and beliefs regarding HIV treatments
* Poor self-efficacy
* Lack of support systems
* Lack of knowledge about HIV and the medications
* Forgetfulness
* Poor patient–provider relationship
* Poor access to drugs (monetary or otherwise)
* Complexity of the regimen (dosing schedule, dietary restrictions, number of medications)
* Medication side effects

How Does the HAART Protocol Address These Factors?

Through the multidisciplinary process, the Protocol provides education concerning HIV, the medications, and their side effects to better enable patients to make informed decisions regarding their therapies. The Protocol process tries to identify barriers to adherence such as mental health issues, lack of support, substance use, homelessness, and then promote resolution of those barriers prior to starting antiretrovirals. HAART should never be thought of as an emergency; a delay of a few weeks in starting HAART to better prepare patients for the needed commitment could mean the difference between success and failure of HAART.

Has the HAART Protocol Been Shown to Impact Adherence?

A preliminary 6-month analysis of medication adherence, as measured through pharmacy refill histories, showed the following results:

6-Month Adherence	Retrospective Control Group (A) n= 288	HAART Protocol Group (B) n= 73	P
Mean Adherence	88%	97%	0.04
≥95%	40%	54%	
≥90%	49%	57%	

Among the 125 patients in Group A and 60 in Group B who had detectable viral loads at baseline, 58% and 77% respectively had undetectable viral loads (<500 copies/mL) at 6 months (p=0.02). These results indicate that patients who completed our clinic's HAART Protocol prior to starting HAART were more likely to adhere to their HAART regimens and have successful viral load response. A subsequent analysis of the effect of the HAART Protocol is under evaluation at this time and results may be available soon.

What Is the Role of Each Discipline Within the HAART Protocol?

The following is a list of each member's responsibilities within this protocol. Each of the disciplines responsible for interviews shall complete a portion of the routing slip to facilitate communication of their findings back to the provider.

I. Provider's Role

1. Refer Patients to the HAART Protocol as Appropriate:
    a. Who is required to go through the Protocol?
        i. HAART-naïve patients
        ii. Patients that have been off of a HAART regimen for 6 months or more.
    b. If your patient is still on medications or has been off them for <6 months, you can put him or her through the "On-HAART" Protocol. On the top

of the HAART Form, cross out "Pre" and write "On" HAART and you can specify which disciplines you would like your patient to see for more in-depth education.

   c. See above for exceptions to the HAART Protocol Process.

2. Complete the HAART Form (**Figure 13A-1**):

   a. Providers should write as much information as possible concerning the patient's antiretroviral history (including what medications were tried, duration on each medication, any side effects or resistance with particular medications). This will enable pharmacy to better evaluate and promote the next ARV regimen to the patient.

   b. Provide any relevant adherence information (i.e. homelessness, drug use, prior non-adherence, etc.).

   c. Suggest a regimen that you are considering the patient start on. If you would like pharmacy to assist with narrowing down the regimen choices, you can suggest a few regimens and pharmacy will discuss all of the pros and cons with the patient and determine what regimen would work best. Having pharmacy discuss all of the medication ins and outs could save you time during your clinic visit, and you can still feel comfortable because you know all of the information is being covered. None of the other disciplines will ever undermine a provider's suggestion or the patient's trust in their provider, but we may suggest alternatives as appropriate and discuss them with the provider when possible. All comments are written on the HAART Protocol routing slip, so it is important to read them every time.

3. Promote the HAART Protocol Process to Your Patients

The HAART Protocol is designed to educate patients and to identify and correct adherence barriers prior to beginning medications, which will ideally increase the patient's ability to adhere to medications, thus slowing the development of resistance. Everyone at Madison Clinic wants to provide good care to our patients and better enable them to succeed, and we feel the HAART Protocol is part of that mission. If a provider undermines or badmouths the protocol to the patient, it can become very difficult to reach patients as they have already tuned out. Remember, HAART is rarely ever an emergency; a few weeks' delay will not make much difference in the outcome of the patients. Failure of therapy because of non-adherence, however, will make a big difference.

4. Do Not Start the HAART Protocol on a Patient's 1st Visit to the Clinic

New patients to clinic are often overwhelmed by a plethora of information coming at them from many directions. Adding the HAART Protocol to that initial chaos may overwhelm patients further and prevent them from retaining the valuable information presented by each of the disciplines.

AACS Forms Management: PreHaart Routing Flowsheet H1515 Sept 2004

Harborview Madison Clinic PreHAART Routing Flowsheet

PATIENT PHONE NUMBER(S)	RECENT CD4 / % DATE	RECENT VL DATE

PRIMARY CARE PROVIDER

PREVIOUS ANTIRETROVIRALS:

PROPOSED REGIMEN (DISCUSSED TREATMENT STUDY PARTICIPATION ☐ YES ☐ NO)

Check any of the following possible barriers to adherence that apply to your patient:

☐ Active substance abuse ☐ Untreated mental illness ☐ Acute situational stressors
☐ Non-belief in antiretrovirals / disease ☐ History of non-adherence ☐ Fear of side effects
☐ Other:

PROVIDER   (PRINT NAME CLEARLY)   DATE

PROVIDER: please give form to front desk so that appointments can be scheduled

PHARMACY   APPOINTMENT DATE / TIME:
EDUCATION CONDUCTED: ☐ SUGGEST HAART
(SEE ORCA)   ☐ SUGGEST DELAY
NAME & SIGNATURE   DATE

SOCIAL WORK / CASE MANAGER ☐ OOC ☐ LAA ☐ NWFC ☐ MAD SW   APPOINTMENT DATE / TIME:
ASSESSMENT CONDUCTED: ☐ SUGGEST HAART   NAME _____
(SEE ORCA)   ☐ SUGGEST DELAY
NAME & SIGNATURE   DATE

NUTRITION   APPOINTMENT DATE / TIME:
EDUCATION CONDUCTED: ☐ SUGGEST HAART
(SEE ORCA)   ☐ SUGGEST DELAY
NAME & SIGNATURE   DATE

FOLLOWUP TRACKING OF APPOINTMENTS SCHEDULED Outcome: **NS** = No-Show, **R** = Rescheduled, **C** = Cancel

Type	DATE / OUTCOME	DATE / OUTCOME	DATE / OUTCOME	DATE / OUTCOME	DATE / OUTCOME
PHARMACY					
NUTRITION					
SOCIAL WORK					

PROVIDER FOLLOW-UP APPT	DATE	LIST FINAL PRESCRIPTIONS & DATE DISPENSED (PHARMACY ONLY)

EDUCATION ON MEDICATIONS RECEIVED
AT TIME OF DISPENSING?
☐ YES ☐ NO   ☐ PATIENT REFUSED   ☐ BROKEN HAART
                                                     REASON_____

PT.NO

NAME

☐ DOB

UW Medicine
Harborview Medical Center – UW Medical Center
University of Washington Physicians
Seattle, Washington
PRE-HAART ROUTING FLOWSHEET

H1515
H1515
H1515 REV SEPT 04

Figure 13A-1. Pre-HAART Routing Flowsheet

5.   Try Not to Schedule All HAART Appointments on One Day

For the same reason as above, patients can get information overload if they are bombarded all in one day by the three disciplines. Spacing out the appointments will allow the patients more time to process the information. The Protocol is flexible, however, and if patients live very far away or can't make it to clinic often enough, exceptions can be made. But they should be exceptions, and not the norm.

II. Patient's Role

1.   Complete all interviews in a timely manner. Six months should not be exceeded between initiation of the Protocol and initiation of therapy. If appointments are missed or canceled, call the clinic at 731-5100 to reschedule.

2.   Ask any and all pertinent questions regarding antiretroviral therapy.

3.   Communicate back to provider any concerns raised during interviews with the other disciplines.

4.   Once started on therapy, communicate quickly back to provider any disconcerting side effects or difficulties maintaining the schedule of medication taking.

III. Front Desk's Role

1.   Give patients a copy of the *"Starting 'HAART' Medications"* to explain the protocol.

2.   Make sure patients have signed Registry paperwork. If they have not, and they should, sign them up.

3.   Notify Carol Glenn that the patient is here so that she can introduce research studies to him or her.

4.   Schedule Pharmacy and Nutrition appointments in EPIC - Schedule an interpreter if needed.

5.   Write patient information on "HAART Clipboard."

6.   Call or page the patient's social worker while the patient is still in clinic so the social worker can schedule the appointment.

   a.   How to identify the appropriate case manager:

   i.   Look at list of assigned case managers

   ii.   Ask if patient is case managed by NWFC

   •   The front desk will schedule the pharmacy and nutrition appointments first and fill in the dates and times on the HAART form as well as the HAART clipboard.

   •   Have the patient sign a release of information before he or she leaves the clinic and attach to HAART routing slip. ROI to be filed in the NWFC ROI book by Jean Aarvig.

- Then fax a copy of the entire HAART Protocol form (including other HAART appointments) to NWFC. This will alert them to the dates of the other HAART appointments. Fax number is 731-3051.
- Once the fax is received, the form will be forwarded to the correct case manager and that case manager will contact the patient to schedule the HAART appointment.

iii. Ask patient if he or she is case managed outside (e.g., Lifelong AIDS Alliance, Consejo, or non-King county)
- Schedule patient with social work. Gerald will review the social work scheduled and identify the patient's outside social worker to finalize the HAART appointment.

iv. If case manager is unknown, page the on-call case manager (pager: 994-4543). If no response, schedule patient with social work. Gerald will review the social work scheduled and identify the patient's social worker to finalize the appointment.

7. Do NOT make the follow-up appointment with provider. Tell patient to make an appointment with his or her provider after the HAART Protocol is complete.

8. Try NOT to schedule all three appointments on one day; it can overwhelm the patient with information. If patient lives far away or has other extenuating circumstances, you CAN schedule them all on one day if you need to.

9. If patients cancel appointments, when they call back, only schedule one appointment at a time with them. When they come in for that appointment, the next one can be scheduled.

IV. Research Coordinator's Role

1. Present and discuss potential studies with patients and their primary care provider.

V. Social Work's Role

1. Assess a patient's motivation, capacity, and opportunity to adhere to HIV medication, which includes exploring:
   a. Patient's beliefs about HIV and meaning attributed to having HIV;
   b. Patient's beliefs about medicines and the meaning the patient attributes to taking HIV medications;
   c. Patient's relationship with his or her medical team;
   d. Practical barriers to adherence; and
   e. Other factors that may put patient at risk for non-adherence (e.g., untreated mental illness, employment, active substance abuse, stress, etc.).

2. Identify potential barriers to successful adherence and offer interventions to reduce those barriers.

3. Promote a patient's participation in decision-making.

VI. Nutritionist's Role

1. Assess a patient's readiness for antiretroviral therapy by exploring:

    a. Weight history and body changes;

    b. Extensive assessment of diet history to determine if clients are eating well and appropriately as required by medications or existing medical conditions;

    c. Current and proposed medication regimens and whether they should be taken with or without food for optimal efficacy;

    d. Presence of any barriers to eating (i.e., no food, no cooking equipment, no money);

    e. Presence of social factors that negatively impact nutritional status (i.e., smoking, substance use, absence of physical activity or exercise);

    f. Longitudinal monitoring of bioelectrical impedance analysis (BIA) for assessment of changes in body muscle mass, fat, and fluid status over time (e.g., monitoring for lipodystrophy changes);

    g. Diets as needed for clients with special nutritional needs such as diabetes, hepatitis, renal compromise; and

    h. Access to a group weight loss class, as indicated.

VII. Pharmacist's Role

1. Assess a patient's knowledge of HIV and the medications used for its treatment. Assessment involves exploring the following areas:

    a. Patient's attitudes towards and motivation to take antiretrovirals;

    b. Patient's understanding of CD4 count and viral load level, and how the medications work within the body;

    c. Patient's understanding of the importance of medication adherence and how non-adherence contributes to resistance development and treatment failure;

    d. Patient's ability to adhere to specific medication-related dietary requirements;

    e. Patient's awareness of potential medication side effects and techniques for monitoring and preventing those side effects;

    f. Patient's drug and alcohol use; and

    g. Patient's current medication and the potential for drug interactions.

2. Provide information that will better enable the patient to take his or her medications appropriately and achieve better clinical outcomes. This includes:

    a. Clearing up any misconceptions identified during the assessment;

    b. Providing written information on all medications along with contact information for pharmacy or Medcon in case he or she experiences worrisome short- or long-term side-effects;

    c. Emphasizing the importance of routine laboratory and clinical monitoring;

    d. Providing strategies for appropriately handling late or missed doses;

    e. Educating patient about the impact of alcohol and drugs in antiretrovirals; and

    f. Educating patient to always consult provider or pharmacist if he or she begins any new medications.

3. Identify potential barriers to medication adherence and offer interventions to reduce those barriers. Interventions routinely offered include:

    a. Encouraging patients to become their own best advocate by ensuring that they always have access to medications (i.e., planning ahead for vacation supplies, keeping a list of their medications that can be provided for hospital admissions if needed);

    b. Identifying all current medications, reviewing the patients' daily schedules, and creating a medication schedule that will fit well within their lifestyle;

    c. Recommending or providing adherence assistance measures (e.g., weekly pill boxes, alarm devices, or pharmacy-assisted mediset program for medication management); and

    d. Recommending appropriate alternatives in cases where drug interactions exist.

4. Review key points prior to dispensing the medications for the first time and telephone patients 1 week after starting therapy or discuss at the 2-week refill to assess for side effects or other problems that could result in non-adherence or discontinuation of therapy.

References

1. Palella FJ, Delaney KM, Moorman AC, et al. Declining morbidity and mortality among patients with advanced human immunodeficiency virus infection. *N Engl J Med.* 1998; 338(13):853–60.

2. Hogg RS, Heath KV, Yip B, et al. Improved survival among HIV-infected individuals following initiation of antiretroviral therapy. *JAMA.* 1998; 279(6):450–4.

3. Valenti WM. Treatment adherence improves outcomes and manages costs. *AIDS Read.* 2001; 11(2):77–80.

4. Bangsberg DR, Perry S, Charlebois ED, et al. Non-adherence to highly active antiretroviral therapy predicts progression to AIDS. *AIDS.* 2001; 15(9):1181–3.

5. Low-Beer S, Yip B, O'Shaughnessy MV, et al. Adherence to triple therapy and viral load response. *J Acquir Immune Defic Syndr.* 2000; 23(4):360–1.

6. Paterson DL, Swindells S, Mohr J, et al. Adherence to protease inhibitor therapy and outcomes in patients with HIV infection. *Ann Intern Med.* 2000; 133(1):21–30.

7. Bangsberg DR, Hecht FM, Charlebois ED, et al. Adherence to protease inhibitors, HIV-1 viral load and development of drug resistance in an indigent population. *AIDS.* 2000; 14(4):357–66.

8. Bartlett JA. Addressing the challenges of adherence. *J Acquir Immune Defic Syndr.* 2002; 29:S2–S10.

9. Gordillo V, Amo Jd, Soriano V, et al. Sociodemographic and psychological variables influencing adherence to antiretroviral therapy. *AIDS.* 1999; 13:1763–9.

10. Martin-Fernandez J, Escobar-Rodriguez I, Campo-Angora M, et al. Evaluation of adherence to highly active antiretroviral therapy. *Arr Intern Med.* 2001; 161(22):2739–40.

11. Nieuwkerk PT, Sprangers MA, Burger DM, et al. Limited patient adherence to highly active antiretroviral therapy for HIV-1 infection in an observational cohort study. *Arr Intern Med.* 2001; 161(16):1962–8.

The HAART Protocol is a guideline for the clinic and was begun to benefit patient care. It is not a hard and fast rule, and exceptions can be made for legitimate reasons. "Because I want to" is not a legitimate reason, nor is it doing patients any favors. The patient who thinks he or she knows everything is often the one who needs the most education. If a provider wishes to deviate from the HAART Protocol, he or she will be asked to discuss the situation with the clinic's Medical Director, Mac Hooton, or Deputy Medical Director, Bob Harrington. Address any other questions or concerns to the HAART/CQI Committee Chairperson, Beth Hykes, by pager.

Helicobacter Pylori Infection

Ji Eun Lee

Peptic ulcer disease (PUD) is one of the most common causes of upper gastrointestinal (GI) bleeding in the United States; an estimated 25 million people are diagnosed with PUD during their lifetimes, and 6500 deaths occur annually due to complications of the disease.[1] Most cases are associated with an infection of *Helicobacter pylori* (*H. pylori*). *H. pylori* infection is the source of 90% of duodenal ulcers and 70% of gastric ulcers.[2] It has also been associated with the development of gastric cancer and mucosa-associated lymphoid tissue (MALT) lymphoma.[1] Therefore, the successful treatment of *H. pylori* infection will have tremendous impact on decreasing the mortality and morbidity associated with PUD.

Indications

1. Identification of patients with PUD or dyspepsia[3]
   a. Abdominal symptoms including dull, gnawing, abdominal ache that occurs on an empty stomach (2–3 hours after meals or in the middle of the night) and is relieved by food or antacids
   b. Other symptoms including weight loss, poor appetite, bloating, burping, nausea, and vomiting
2. Indications for *H. pylori* testing[3–5]
   a. *H. pylori* testing is indicated for patients with:
      i. Active PUD
      ii. History of documented PUD
      iii. Uninvestigated dyspepsia

iv. Gastric mucosa-associated lymphoid tissue (MALT) lymphoma

v. High risk of gastric cancer

These patients should only be tested if there is intention to treat if the test results confirm infection.

Management

1. Obtain medication allergy history.

2. Obtain complete medication history, including current or recent use of any anti-secretory agents [proton pump inhibitors (PPI) or histamine-2 receptor antagonists (H2RA)].

3. Confirm *H. pylori* infection.[5,6] Patients suspected of *H. pylori* infection should be given a diagnostic test for positive confirmation of infection before initiating treatment. Currently, there is no single gold standard diagnostic test of *H. pylori* infection; therefore, the choice of diagnostic test depends on patient presentation and history. Test methods include serological, urea breath, stool antigen, and the more invasive endoscopic tests.

4. Review local antibiotic resistance of clarithromycin and metronidazole. There is great variability in drug resistance to clarithromycin and metronidazole throughout the country and around the world. The use of antibiotics with high resistance may decrease efficacy of the eradication regimen by up to 20%.[7] Therefore, it is important to review local resistance patterns before initiating an eradication regimen.

5. Pharmacologic treatments[8–10]

   a. First-line treatment: PPI-based triple regimen

   PPI bid + clarithromycin 500 mg bid + amoxicillin 1000 mg bid for 10–14 days

   or

   For patients with penicillin allergy:

   PPI bid + clarithromycin 500 mg bid + metronidazole 500 mg bid for 10–14 days

   The PPI-based triple regimen with two antibiotics has demonstrated an eradication rate of 78–85%.[9] Each of the PPIs has similar efficacy rates; therefore, the choice of an agent is dependent on cost and individual patient tolerability. Currently, there is no firm consensus on the appropriate length of therapy. Some studies suggest that longer treatment duration of 10–14 days may have higher eradication rates as compared to 7-day therapy.[8]

   b. Second-line treatment: quadruple regimen

   PPI bid + bismuth subsalicylate 525 mg qid + metronidazole 500 mg tid

+ tetracycline 500 mg qid for 10–14 days

Second-line therapy is indicated and should be initiated immediately when post-eradication testing reveals failure of the first-line regimen. If failure was due to non-adherence of first-line therapy, attempt another course of first-line treatment after counseling patient about the importance of completing the regimen. The quadruple regimen with PPI, bismuth, and two antibiotics has been shown to be 81–88% effective in eradicating the infection.[9] Compared to the first-line regimen, there is greater risk for decreased medication adherence and poor tolerability due to increased side-effect potential and a more complex dosing schedule.

c. Third-line treatments[7,10,11]

Patients who have failed two eradication regimens should be referred to a gastroenterologist. Endoscopy with biopsy and culture is recommended in these patients to assist in selection of further treatments. Additional PPI-based triple and quadruple combinations with alternative antibiotics have been studied with levofloxacin, moxifloxacin, tinidazole, rifabutin, and azithromycin with substantial cure rates. Currently, these antibiotics are indicated only in third-line regimens, but further clinical trials may demonstrate their usefulness in first- and second-line treatments.

6. Post-treatment follow-up[5,9]

a. Eradication of *H. pylori* should be verified in complicated PUD, persistent symptoms after initial course of *H. pylori* eradication therapy, gastric MALT lymphoma, and early gastric cancer. Additionally, symptom resolution does not necessarily indicate *H. pylori* eradication; therefore, follow-up confirmation testing is useful. Post-treatment eradication verification of *H. pylori* can be done by urea breath test, stool antigen test, or endoscopy with biopsy. The test should be performed at least 4 weeks after completing a treatment regimen and at least 1–2 weeks after discontinuing all anti-secretory medications such as PPIs or H2RAs.

b. Patients with active or complicated PUD may require maintenance therapy with a PPI for an additional 4–8 weeks for ulcer healing. In patients with uncomplicated ulcers or dyspepsia, maintenance therapy is not recommended.

c. Instruct patient to return for additional care if returning or worsening dyspepsia symptoms and/or alarm symptoms (unexplained weight loss, dysphagia, vomiting, unexplained bleeding) occur. Patients should be educated about non-pharmacologic treatments for dyspepsia/GERD.

Goals of Therapy

1. Eradicate *H. pylori* with simple, cost-effective, well-tolerated, pharmacologic regimens.
2. Reduce the risk of complicated PUD or development of gastric MALT lymphoma or gastric cancer.

Clinical Pharmacy Goals

1. Ensure appropriate eradication treatment regimen to prevent treatment failures.
2. Educate patients about the importance of compliance, proper administration, and potential adverse reactions with selected treatment regimens.
3. Educate patients about preventative measures for dyspepsia symptoms.
4. Educate patients to seek additional care in case of worsening or returning symptoms and/or alarm symptoms.

Outcome Measures

1. Process measures: Decreased incidence of eradication treatment failure; antibacterial resistance rates; patient adherence to prescribed therapy.
2. Health outcome measures: Reduced peptic ulcer complications (GI bleed, gastric MALT lymphoma, gastric cancer).

Patient Information Resources

1. National Digestive Diseases Information Clearinghouse: http:// digestive.niddk.nih.gov/ddiseases/pubs/hpylori
2. UpToDate: http://patients.uptodate.com/topic.asp?file=digestiv/8187
3. Helicobacter Foundation: http://www.helico.com
4. Centers for Disease Control and Prevention: http://www.cdc.gov/ncidod/ dbmd/diseaseinfo/hpylori_g.htm
5. Medline Plus: http://www.nlm.nih.gov/medlineplus/pepticulcer.html

CASE STUDY

S: A 52-yo female with a 6-month history of increasing stomach pain is diagnosed with a gastric ulcer. Recent endoscopy reveals presence of *H. pylori* in the stomach. Patient was prescribed triple regimen with lansoprazole, amoxicillin, and clarithromycin. After 2 days of therapy, patient discontinued her regimen due to intolerable bad taste in her mouth and diarrhea. Patient would like an alternative regimen that she can better tolerate.

Allergies: NKDA

Current medications:

Hydrochlorothiazide 25 mg daily

Lisinopril 20 mg daily

Naproxen 500 mg q 12 h

Acetaminophen 500 mg q 6 h prn

Lansoprazole 30 mg bid x 10 days

Amoxicillin 1 g bid x 10 days

Clarithromycin 500 mg bid x 10 days

PMH: Hypertension

Osteoarthritis

FH: Non-contributory

SH: Tobacco: 1 ppd x 30 years

Alcohol: 1 beer daily

Drinks 1 cup of coffee every morning

O: BP 136/76, HR 67 bpm, RR 18, T 36.7°C

Weight: 74 kg

General: Alert, oriented, NAD

HEENT: PERRLA

Ext: WNL

Neuro: AO x 3

(+) guaiac – prior to endoscopy

Pathology: Biopsy (genta stain): (+) *H. pylori*

Diagnosis: *H. pylori* with gastric ulcer

Labs: WNL

A/P:

1. Patient is experiencing intolerable side effects from *H. pylori* regimen with clarithromycin, lansoprazole, and amoxicillin. *Of all the PPIs, lansoprazole has the highest rate of diarrhea; therefore, it is an option to change to another agent in the class to decrease side effects. The intolerance to clarithromycin is more difficult to solve. If the patient is willing to tolerate the bad taste for 8 more days, her current regimen should be continued with a change in her PPI. If the patient adamantly refuses to take clarithromycin, she should be changed to the quadruple regimen, which has more complex dosing and a similar risk of undesirable side effects. In addition, due to her chronic alcohol use, metronidazole would be contraindicated for this patient. If the patient is unwilling to take her clarithromycin and is willing to stop drinking for the next 2 weeks, then her regimen can be changed to the recommended quadruple regimen.*

2. Change regimen to bismuth subsalicylate 525 mg qid, metronidazole 500 mg tid, tetracycline 500 mg qid, and pantoprazole 40 mg bid for 10 days. *The patient needs to be counseled on the importance of completing the therapy to decrease risk of resistance and to eradicate the infection. She also needs education about nonpharmacologic therapy to prevent dyspepsia symptoms.*

3. Counsel patient to abstain from alcohol consumption during therapy and to take PPI 30 minutes to 1 hour prior to meals (breakfast/dinner or lunch/dinner if no breakfast).

4. Discontinue naproxen. Increase acetaminophen up to 1 g q 6 h prn to control arthritis pain if necessary. *Patient needs to discontinue naproxen to decrease risk of worsening gastric ulcer.*

   Counsel patient on the importance of smoking cessation. Cigarette use may alter healing and also is a risk factor for PUD.

5. Continue pantoprazole 40 mg daily for 8 weeks after completion of *H. pylori* treatment. *Since the patient has newly diagnosed gastric ulcer, she would need to take a PPI for 8 weeks after completion of* H. pylori *treatment. If the patient's symptoms improve, confirmation of eradication of* H. pylori *is not necessary. If confirmation is needed, eradication can be confirmed with urea breath test or stool antigen test.*

References

1. ASHP therapeutic position statement on the identification and treatment of *helicobacter pylori*-associated peptic ulcer disease in adults. *Am J Health-Syst Pharm.* 2001; 58(4):331–7.

2. Talley NJ, Vakil NB, Moayyedi P. American gastroenterological association technical review on the evaluation of dyspepsia. *Gastroenterology.* 2005; 129:1756–80.

3. Talley NJ, Vakil N. Guidelines for the management of dyspepsia. *Am J Gastroenterol.* 2005; 100:2324–37.

4. Howden CW, Hunt RH. Guidelines for the management of Helicobacter pylori infection. *Am J Gastroenterol.* 1998; 93(12):2330–8.

5. Peterson WL, Fendrick AM, Cave DR, et al. Helicobacter pylori—related disease. *Arch Intern Med.* 2000; 160:1285–91.

6. Ong SP, Duggan A. Eradication of Helicobacter pylori in clinical situations. *Clin Exp Med.* 2004; 3:30–8.

7. Calvet X. Helicobacter pylori infection: treatment options. *Digestion.* 2006; 73(s1):119–28.

8. Bytzer P, O'Morain C. Treatment of Helicobacter pylori. *Helicobacter.* 2003; 10:S40–6.

9. Malfertheiner P, Mergraud F, O'Morain C, et al. Current concepts in the management of Helicobacter pylori infection—The Maastricht 2-2000 consensus report. *Aliment Pharmacol Ther.* 2002; 6:167–80.

10. Stable BE, Smith BR, Weeks DL. Helicobacter pylori infection and surgical disease—part I. *Curr Probl Surg.* 2005; 42:756–89.

11. Gisbert JP, Pajares JM. Helicobacter pylori "rescue" therapy after failure of two eradication treatments. *Helicobacter.* 2005; 10:363–72.

Chronic Non-Malignant Pain

Carrie L. Yuan

Various chronic pain syndromes account for three of the top ten reasons for visits to physician offices.[1] Physicians are under increasing pressure to address issues surrounding pain, especially with organizations such as the Joint Commission® stating that patients have a right to pain assessment and treatment.[2] Because medical treatment of chronic pain is perhaps the most frequently utilized modality, pharmacists are in an excellent position to lend their expertise to management of this increasingly common yet often complicated disorder.

Indications

Identification of Patients with Chronic Non-Malignant Pain

1. Patients with non-malignant pain, which is chronic in nature (duration >3 months). The etiologies of non-malignant pain syndromes are numerous and include, but are not limited to, osteoarthritis/degenerative joint disease, back pain, neuropathic pain, and fibromyalgia.

Identification of Patients to Be Managed with Opioids

1. Patients with pain refractory to non-opioid medications who have tried and failed multiple treatment modalities.

2. The decision to treat a patient with opioids for chronic pain should be multi-disciplinary and, when indicated, include consultation with pharmacists, physical therapists, social workers, mental health providers, and others.

Management

Non-Opioid Medications

Every effort is made to manage chronic pain with non-opioid medications, including acetaminophen and non-steroidal anti-inflammatory drugs (NSAIDs). Medications such as tricyclic antidepressants, gabapentin, and other anticonvulsants are useful for neuropathic pain. Non-opioid medications are often used in conjunction with opioids in an attempt to minimize opioid doses.

Opioids

Evidence demonstrating the effectiveness of long-term opioids for chronic non-malignant pain is limited (Level IV) at best.[3-5] Despite the lack of conclusive data, providers are turning to opioids for patients whose pain remains refractory to other interventions. Long-acting opioids are preferred for most patients when opioids are prescribed for long-term management of chronic pain. Opioids with a long half-life (e.g., methadone) or controlled-release formulation (e.g., MS Contin®) have a lower abuse potential and street value as compared to the highly reinforcing characteristics of high-peaking, rapid-onset, short-acting opioids (e.g., hydromorphone, oxycodone).[6] It is, however, important to note that all opioids have the potential for abuse. Many providers choose not to prescribe the long-acting oxycodone formulation (OxyContin®), which has gained notoriety for its abuse potential, and in some areas of the country demands a street value as high as $2.50 per milligram.[7] Short-acting opioids may be appropriate for some patients, such as those with pain that is chronic in duration but not persistent. Opioids should be discontinued if satisfactory analgesia and improvement in functionality are not achieved or if adverse effects are intolerable.

Prescribers are responsible for regular review of patients' chronic pain therapy, including review of the medical diagnoses, any psychiatric diagnoses, assessment of opioid and/or non-opioid medications with or without non-medical interventions such as physical therapy, and pre- and post-intervention assessment of pain scores and functional levels. Routine assessment of the "4 As"—analgesia, activity, aberrant behavior, and adverse effects—can help to direct therapy.

In our facility, the clinical pharmacy specialists maintain an electronic registry of patients receiving long-term opioids for chronic pain. This registry assists prescribers by tracking prescription fill dates and improving practice efficiency. In addition to prescription data, pharmacists use the registry to track clinical data such as pain scores, results of urine toxicology screens, and any breaches of the opioid agreement. Although the registry is currently only accessible by pharmacists, the goal is to provide access within the medical center to facilitate continuity of care among primary, specialty, and acute care providers.

Opioid Agreements

An opioid agreement (also known as a "contract") (**Appendix 15-1**) is a formal and explicit written agreement between prescriber and patient, outlining the terms of use of opioids for chronic pain. Opponents of the opioid agreement view it as paternalistic, punitive, and intimidating; some suggest it promotes pseudo-addictive behavior. The most frequently cited justifications for opioid agreements are in promoting patient adherence, providing informed consent, minimizing legal risk, and improving practice efficiency. Although opioid agreement use is popular, there is minimal empirical evidence for the effectiveness of agreements in achieving their intended objectives.[8] The use of opioid agreements may be an expression of the uncertainty of the real benefits and risks of long-term opioid therapy for chronic non-malignant pain, a topic that is widely debated and highly controversial.[5,8]

Despite unproven effectiveness of opioid agreements, most prescribers in our institution have decided to require all patients receiving opioids on a chronic basis to sign an agreement and informed consent (**Appendix 15-2**). This removes personal bias and the need for judgment on the part of the prescriber to decide or predict which patients have the potential for aberrant drug-taking behavior. An informed consent serves to make patients aware of the potential for serious adverse effects from opioids (e.g., physical dependence or abuse, hyperalgia, cardiopulmonary toxicity) and to discuss medically acceptable alternatives to opioids.

Goals of Therapy

1. Provide clinically appropriate, comprehensive, considerate, and respectful care that accepts and acts upon patients' report of pain.
2. Engage patients in establishing and achieving self-management goals that reduce pain and improve functional status.

Clinical Pharmacy Goals

1. Provide recommendations to providers with regard to drug and dose selection.
2. Educate patients on medications used to treat chronic pain, and assist patients in forming realistic expectations of pain relief provided by medications.
3. Reduce the risk of inappropriate prescribing of opioids and minimize the risk of illegal diversion.

Outcome Measures

Due to the subjective nature of chronic pain, the implementation of processes for assessment and tracking of goals of therapy and clinical outcomes is a challenging area that requires more study and attention. Some suggested outcome measures are:

1. Surrogate clinical markers: Patient's report of pain pre- and post-intervention.

2. Health outcome measures: Change in functional status or ability to perform activities of daily living.

Patient Information Resources

1. Chronic Pain Information Page from the National Institutes of Health: http://www.ninds.nih.gov/disorders/chronic_pain/chronic_pain.htm

2. Information about chronic pain medicines from the American Academy of Family Physicians: http://familydoctor.org/122.xml

3. Managing chronic pain: http://www.fda.gov/FDAC/features/2004/204_pain.html

References

1. Hing E, Cherry DK, Woodwell DA, et al. National Ambulatory Medical Care Survey: 2004 Summary. Advanced Data 2006; 374:1–34. Available at http://www.cdc.gov/nchs/data/ad/ad374.pdf. Accessed February 24, 2007.

2. The Joint Commission News Room, Health Care Issues. Available at http://www.jointcommission.org/NewsRoom/health_care_issues.htm. Accessed February 26, 2007.

3. Chou R. Drug Class Review on Long-Acting Opioid Analgesics. Final Report 2006. Available at http://www.ohsu.edu/drugeffectiveness/reports/final.cfm. Accessed February 26, 2007.

4. Martell BA, O'Connor PG, Kerns RD, et al. Systematic review: opioid treatment for chronic back pain: prevalence, efficacy, and association with addiction. *Ann Intern Med.* 2007; 146:116–27.

5. Trescot AM, Boswell MV, Atluri SL, et al. Opioid guidelines in the management of chronic non-cancer pain. *Pain Physician.* 2006; 9:1–40.

6. Brookoff D. Abuse potential of various opioid medications. *J Gen Intern Med.* 1993; 8:688–90.

7. U.S. DEA Briefs and Backgrounds, Drugs and Drug Abuse, State Factsheets – Kentucky. Available at http://www.usdoj.gov/dea/pubs/states/kentucky2006.html. Accessed February 24, 2007.

8. Arnold RA, Han PJK, Seltzer D. Opioid contracts in chronic nonmalignant pain management: objectives and uncertainties. *Am J Med.* 2006; 119:292–6.

Appendix 15-1: Draft Chronic Pain Contract

HMC WILL PROVIDE CONTROLLED SUBSTANCE MEDICATIONS TO YOU
ONLY IF YOU ARE IN AGREEMENT WITH THE FOLLOWING STIPULATIONS:

Check (✓) Box

☐ I agree to obtain all prescriptions for controlled substance medications only from HMC pharmacy during the hours of 0800 – 2200.

☐ I agree to take the controlled substance medication only as prescribed by my physician.

☐ I agree to follow the advice of HMC physicians regarding the dose and plan of care while using controlled substance medications.

☐ I am responsible for the controlled substance medications prescribed to me. I am aware my prescription will not be replaced if lost, misplaced, stolen, or if "I run out early".

☐ My use of controlled substance medications will be reassessed by my provider at least every 3-4 months, or sooner as stated by the provider.

☐ If I fail to keep an appointment my prescription may not be refilled. I will keep all appointments with my provider, chemical dependency counselor, and/or psychiatrist.

☐ I will provide a <u>urine drug test</u> at the request of the HMC medical staff at any time it is requested. If the test is positive for illicit drugs or a non-prescribed controlled substance, the Agreement for Treatment of Pain with a Controlled Substance may be terminated.

☐ If I sell my controlled substance medications, the Agreement for Treatment of Pain with a Controlled Substance will be terminated.

☐ I understand abusive behavior toward staff or other patients will not be tolerated and will result in termination of the Agreement for Treatment of Pain with a Controlled Substance.

☐ If I forge a prescription or sell the prescribed controlled substance, the Agreement for Treatment of Pain with a Controlled Substance will be terminated **and the police will be notified**.

☐ I agree to inform my provider of my complete and honest personal drug history, including the drug history of anyone in my family.

☐ For women: If I plan to become pregnant or believe that I have become pregnant while taking a controlled substance medication, I will immediately notify my provider.

☐ I understand that the main goals of treatment with chronic controlled substance medications are to reduce pain **and** improve my overall function. I agree to help myself reach these goals by following healthy lifestyles. This includes exercising, proper nutrition and avoiding alcohol, illicit drugs and tobacco.

_____   _____
PATIENT SIGNATURE   *DATE & TIME*

_____   _____
PHYSICIAN SIGNATURE   *DATE & TIME*

PT.NO

NAME   Place EPIC Label Within Box

DOB

UW Medicine
Harborview Medical Center – UW Medical Center
University of Washington Physicians
Seattle, Washington
**AGREEMENT FOR THE USE OF CONTROLLED
SUBSTANCE MEDICATIONS**

U2127

UH2127 REV JAN 06

PATIENT CARE DOCUMENTATION – BROWN

Appendix 15-2: Draft Chronic Pain Informed Consent

I hereby authorize Dr. _____ and such assistants as may be designated to manage and treat my diagnosis and/or condition of persistent pain with controlled substances.

_____
(NAME OF PATIENT)

WE HAVE DISCUSSED POTENTIAL SIDE EFFECTS AND RISKS OF CONTROLLED SUBSTANCES, INCLUDING:

- ❑ Sleepiness, confusion, difficulty thinking, nausea, vomiting, constipation, difficulty breathing, shortness of breath, wheezing, rash, and itching.
- ❑ Potential for allergic reaction.
- ❑ Potential for interaction with other medications (increasing effects or side effects of drugs taken together).
- ❑ Potential for dependence (after the body adjusts to these medications, they cannot be stopped suddenly without causing physical symptoms).
- ❑ Potential for withdrawal (stopping medications abruptly may cause nausea, vomiting, abdominal pain, sweating, aching, abnormal heartbeat or other symptoms that can be life threatening; medication changes should be under provider supervision).
- ❑ Potential for addiction (compulsive drug use not related to pain relief).
- ❑ Potential for impaired judgment and/or motor skills (driving or operating machinery may be hazardous due to effects on the brain and nerves)
- ❑ Long-term adverse consequences of chronic opioid use are unclear, but may include reduced fertility, sex drive. Long-term use may also result in immunosuppressive and opioid-induced abnormal pain sensitivity.
- ❑ Other: _____

OTHER INFORMATION:

Alternatives to the above treatment plan, which may include doing nothing at all, are:

_____

If I choose to go without the recommended care and treatment plan recommended by my physician, I understand that I may experience physical and other problems, such as:

_____

which have been explained to me and that I have had an opportunity to ask questions and have them answered to my satisfaction.

IF THIS FORM ACCURATELY REPRESENTS OUR DISCUSSION, AND IF YOU ARE SATISFIED WITH THE EXPLANATION GIVEN, YOU MUST SIGN THIS DOCUMENT INDICATING YOUR CONSENT TO THE USE OF CONTROLLED SUBSTANCES IN TREATING YOUR INTRACTABLE PAIN PRIOR TO COMMENCING THE TREATMENT.

HEALTH CARE PROVIDER OBTAINING CONSENT (NAME & INITIAL)	SIGNATURE OF PERSON GIVING CONSENT
DATE SIGNED	TIME ❑ A.M. ❑ P.M.	RELATIONSHIP TO PATIENT (IF APPLICABLE)
❑ PLEASE CHECK IF THIS IS A TELEPHONE CONSENT. THIS CONSENT WILL BE PERMANENTLY FILED IN THE PATIENT'S MEDICAL RECORD	

PT.NO		UW Medicine
		Harborview Medical Center – UW Medical Center
		University of Washington Physicians
		Seattle, Washington
NAME	Place EPIC Label Within Box	**INFORMED CONSENT FOR TREATMENT OF**
		INTRACTABLE PAIN WITH A CONTROLLED SUBSTANCE
DOB		*U2126*
		UH2126 REV JAN 06

CONSENT — GRAY

Orthopedic Pain Management

Myrna Romack, Stephen Strockbine   **CHAPTER**
16

With busy surgical practices and little time available to spend in a clinic, orthopedic surgeons are challenged to manage post-surgical pain. The orthopedic pharmacy service manages outpatient pain medications between clinic visits and when consulted by providers. Service is provided to three orthopedic trauma teams and hand, foot, and ankle as well as spine clinics with 20 attending physicians and 50 fellows and residents. The clinical pharmacy specialists have DEA numbers and prescriptive authority (see **Appendix 16-1**) for narcotics, including CIIs. Therefore, the team is able to provide prompt response to patient requests and concerns. By providing medication between visits and triaging questions and concerns, pharmacists can minimize emergency department visits and remove the burden of pain management from surgeons. Because pharmacists are the sole providers of medication outside of clinic visits, the potential for drug diversion and duplication is minimized.

Indications

Patients treated by orthopedic surgeons status post-orthopedic trauma and/or orthopedic surgery who need pain management services. This management may involve the tapering of narcotics, adjustments for increased pain and the balance between long-acting and short-acting agents, treatment of neuropathic pain, substitution of non-narcotic medications and adjuncts, and the avoidance of adverse drug reactions. Because Harborview is the only Level 1 trauma center for a four-state region, pain management services are routinely provided to patients who reside far from the medical center. Clinical pharmacy specialists provide the majority of this work over the telephone.

Management

Narcotic Analgesics

1. Provide adequate and consistent pain management using narcotic analgesics dosed in appropriate amounts and intervals to "bridge" a patient to the next orthopedic clinic visit. This may require adjustments in long- and short-acting opiates or increasing the total dose of narcotics. Long-acting agents are used for a short period of time to moderate the use of short-acting agents (e.g., consider oxycodone SR if doses of oxycodone 5 mg exceed 12 tablets/day).

2. Gradually decrease the daily dose of narcotic analgesics, as appropriate. The goal is to provide a maximum 1-month supply of Schedule II narcotic therapy followed by 1 month of Schedule III–V therapy and subsequently transition to non-narcotic medication as needed.

Non-Narcotic Medications

It is important to promote the use of non-narcotic analgesics [e.g., acetaminophen and nonsteroidal anti-inflammatory drugs (NSAIDs)], adjunctive therapies (e.g., antihistamines), and agents to prevent side effects (e.g., stool softeners and stimulant laxatives; bulk laxatives are not appropriate for opiate-induced constipation). Medications used to treat neuropathic pain (e.g., gabapentin, tricyclic antidepressants) are also prescribed based on patient presentation and diagnostic studies. Labs are reviewed at baseline and at appropriate intervals, then interpreted; pharmacotherapy is adjusted as necessary.

Goals of Therapy

1. Improve patient's report of pain.
2. Improve patient's functional status.
3. Taper narcotic medication to baseline.
4. Manage adverse effects.

Clinical Pharmacy Goals

1. Improve quality of care through continuity of pain management from inpatient through discharge to outpatient care.
2. Identify patients with pain-related problems.
3. Ensure utilization of appropriate pharmacotherapy.
4. Educate patients, families, providers, and staff about medications and their use in pain management.
5. Minimize emergency department visits strictly for pain medication-related issues.

6. Relieve physicians from clinic visits dealing strictly with pain medication issues.

7. Minimize potential for narcotic diversion/duplication because all narcotic analgesic prescriptions and issues outside of clinic visits are managed by the clinical pharmacy specialists.

8. Refer patients with chronic pain to primary care for inclusion in the pain registry and a pain contract (see Chapter 15, Appendix 15-1).

9. After consultation with orthopedic provider, refer patients with complex or unresolved pain to a pain management clinic.

Outcome Measures

1. Care process measures: Provider assessment; functional status.

2. Surrogate clinical markers: Patient report of pain or other symptoms using rating scales.

3. Health outcome measures: Reduction in emergency department and physician visits strictly for pain medication-related issues.

Patient Information Resources

1. International Association for the Study of Pain: http://www.iasp-pain.org

2. The National Academy of Sciences and the Institute of Medicine: http://www.nationalacademies.org

3. The National Institutes of Health: http://www.nih.gov

4. The National Institute for Clinical Excellence: http://www.nice.org.uk

5. The National Health and Medical Research Council of Australia: http://www.painmgmt.usyd.edu.au/acutepain.html

CASE STUDY

S: 41-year-old male 3 weeks status post open reduction and internal fixation of acetabular fracture sustained in work-related accident presents to clinic stating he needs more oxycodone. He states that he is using medication as originally prescribed but is having uncontrolled pain, which he rates as 7/10. He describes some pain at fracture site but states that more bothersome is a burning and tingling sensation in his foot. Past medical history negative except for tobacco use.

NKDA

Current medications:

Oxycodone 5 mg tablets 1–3 q 4 hours prn pain

Docusate

Senna

O: Last prescription of oxycodone 5 mg tablets #150 Sig: 1–3 q 4 hours prn pain received 7 days ago. On discharge from the hospital 2 weeks prior, he received MS Contin 15 mg #14 to take one tablet every 12 hours and oxycodone 5 mg #150 1–4 q 3 hours prn pain.

A: Patient is using more narcotic medication than prescribed and has increased usage. Patient is experiencing neuropathic pain as indicated by description of burning and tingling pain.

P:

1. Educated patient regarding the causes of his two different types of pain and the most appropriate therapy for each. *Narcotics in general are not good modulators of neuropathic pain, with the possible exception of methadone. His fracture/surgical pain is resolving and so it is anticipated that narcotic medication will be able to be tapered; no further long-acting medication should be needed at this point.*

2. Continue oxycodone to be taken at a decreasing dosage of one less tablet daily.

3. Add acetaminophen 500 mg 1–2 q 6h prn pain; maximum 4000 mg per day.

4. Start gabapentin 300 mg daily to treat neuropathic pain. Increase dose by 300 mg per day until relief of pain, excess sedation, or 3600 mg per day. *Alternatively could use a tricyclic antidepressant such as amitriptyline or nortriptyline to start.*

5. Instructed pt to call with any problems or concerns or when nearing end of supply of either medication.

Bibliography

1. Department of Labor and Industries Attending Doctors Handbook, Section 4. Available at: www.LNI.wa.gov/IPUB/252-004-000.pdf Accessed November 27, 2006.

2. *Essential elements of effective pain management: a standards-based approach.* Oakbrook, IL: Joint Commission Resources; 2001.

3. Holdcroft A, Power I. Recent developments: management of pain. *BMJ.* 2003; 326(7390):635–9.

4. U.S. Department of Justice. Mid-Level Practitioners Authorization by State. Available at: http://www.deadiversion.usdoj.gov/drugreg/practioners/index.html. Accessed May 16, 2007.

Appendix 16-1: HMC Pharmacist Prescriptive Authority Protocol for Pain Management

HARBORVIEW MEDICAL CENTER

PHARMACIST PRESCRIPTIVE AUTHORITY PROTOCOL FOR PAIN MANAGEMENT

GOAL: To enable the pharmacists at Harborview Medical Center (HMC) orthopedic clinic to provide continuity of care for patients by:

1. Providing adequate and consistent pain management through the use of narcotic analgesics dosed in appropriate amounts and intervals to get a patient to the next clinic visit where he or she can be reassessed or for a pre-planned (with the provider) time period.

2. Promoting and providing adequate pain management through the use of non-narcotic analgesics and adjunctive therapy, when appropriate.

3. Gradually decreasing daily dosage of narcotic analgesics, when appropriate. In general, aim for 1 month maximum of Schedule II narcotics followed by 1 month maximum of Schedule III–V narcotics post orthopedic injury or surgery. This may vary depending on the individual patient.

4. Adhering to published pain management guidelines such as those by JCAHO.

   By providing this service, we will be able to improve drug-dosing consistency, improve quality of care, and free providers' time from tasks that can be completed by appropriately trained pharmacists.

INCLUSIONS: The orthopedic clinic pharmacists are granted the authority to initiate or modify pain medication regimens for patients cared for by providers of the orthopedic clinic at HMC with the above goals in mind. Medications include narcotic analgesics, non-narcotic analgesics such as nonsteroidal anti-inflammatory drugs or acetaminophen, tricyclic antidepressants, or gabapentin only to treat nerve pain, and adjunctive agents such as antihistamines, antiemetics, and stool softeners/laxatives.

Muscle relaxants, benzodiazepines, and zolpidem cannot be prescribed by the pharmacist without approval by a provider.

PROCEDURES:

1. For each encounter, the pharmacist will review the patient's medical record and pharmacy profile to determine the injury or procedure performed, medication history, and other relevant medical history.

2. The pharmacist will discuss with the patient or his or her agent medication use, its effect, and any adverse effects.

3. The pharmacist will develop a pain medication plan for the patient with input from his or her provider if necessary.

   a. If patient has been adherent to medication instructions and is adequately controlled, the pharmacist will prescribe medication as above with the attempt to lessen overall narcotic usage through change to lower dosage or lower potency agent or to non-narcotic agent.

   b. If patient has taken more medication than prescribed, the pharmacist will determine the reason and take appropriate action. Possible examples include:

      i. Original prescription not adequate—adjust to control pain, then taper.

      ii. Increased pain due to infection or re-injury—advise patient to be seen by provider to evaluate.

      iii. Patient does not understand directions or intent of medication.

      iv. Lost medication—replace once in a lifetime.

      v. Abuse or diversion—contact provider.

4. Pharmacist will evaluate any adverse effects

   a. If event can be managed by medication change, discontinuation, or by prescribing an adjunctive medication, then pharmacist will take appropriate action. Examples include:

      i. Itching, but no rash with narcotic—add antihistamine, decrease narcotic intake.

      ii. Nausea/vomiting with narcotic—decrease dosage, change drug, add anti-emetic.

      iii. Minor allergic reaction (rash)—discontinue agent, change drug, add antihistamine.

      iv. Constipation—encourage clear liquids, fruits, and vegetables; ensure stool softener use; add laxative if necessary.

      v. Gastrointestinal upset with NSAID—change to different agent; refer to primary care or emergency if suspect serious GI adverse effect.

   b. If event is more serious, refer for medical assessment. Examples:

      i. Hives or anaphylactic reaction—911 or emergency room.

      ii. Unresolved constipation after above tried or suspected bowel obstruction—refer for medical assessment.

DOCUMENTATION: All pharmacist activities will be recorded in the patient's medical record as a progress note or dictated note.

QUALITY ASSURANCE: Periodic evaluation of pharmacist activities will be performed.

Osteoarthritis

Vicki DeCaro, Mary Sturgeleski Kelly, Elaine Pappas

Osteoarthritis (OA) is the most common form of arthritis in the United States, affecting 20.7 million adults.[1] It impacts nearly 50% of individuals over the age of 65, and almost everyone over the age of 75. Also known as degenerative joint disease, it is a leading cause of disability, second only to cardiovascular disease.[2] Although there is no known cure for OA, pharmacists in collaboration with other health care providers can help design a medication regimen to reduce pain, maintain and/or improve joint mobility, and improve quality of life.

Indications

Patients presenting with one or more of the following symptoms or a diagnosis of osteoarthritis:

1. Joint pain (pain involving one or only a few joints). Typical joints include spine, hip, hands (distal) and knee.[3]
2. Joint stiffness (usually occurring in the morning and resolving within 30 minutes, or occurring with mild-to-moderate activity).[3]
3. Joint enlargement or deformity (evidence of disease progression).[3]

Management

Non-Pharmacologic Treatment

Non-pharmacologic therapy is the foundation of osteoarthritis management. It should be initiated before, or simultaneously with, the initiation of pharmacologic therapy.[2,3] Many of these interventions require referral to other health care disciplines (e.g., nutrition, physical therapy, occupational therapy). Aspects of non-pharmacologic therapy include:

1. Patient education

2. Weight loss (if the patient is overweight) through the use of dietary intervention and a structured weight-loss program. Maintaining an appropriate body weight may be the single most important factor in preventing the occurrence of OA in weight-bearing joints.[4]

3. Self-management programs (e.g., Arthritis Foundation Self-Help Program)[5]

4. Personalized social support through telephone contact

5. Physical therapy range-of-motion exercises

6. Muscle-strengthening exercises

7. Assistive devices for ambulation

8. Patellar taping

9. Appropriate footwear

10. Lateral-wedged insoles

11. Occupational therapy

12. Joint protection and rest

13. Assistive devices for daily living

14. Smoking cessation

Pharmacologic Treatment

Initial pharmacologic treatment for mild to moderate pain should begin with topical analgesics or acetaminophen. If inflammation is present or there is no response to these agents, NSAID (non-steroidal anti-inflammatory drug) therapy may be introduced.[2] Upon initiation of pharmacologic therapy, non-pharmacologic treatments should be continued as these regimens often provide as much relief as pharmacologic therapy.

1. Topical analgesics[2,3]

   a. Capsaicin 0.025% or 0.075% cream (start with lower strength)

      i. Notify patient that it may take up to 2 weeks to experience full benefit and to use on a regular basis for best results.

      ii. Counsel patients that a local burning sensation is common, to wash hands after each application, and to avoid contact with the eyes and mucous membranes.

2. Oral analgesics[2,3]

   a. Acetaminophen

      i. First-line therapy due to its relative safety, efficacy, and lower cost compared to NSAIDs.

- May initiate at higher dosage (e.g., 1 gram qid) and taper down as pain subsides and becomes better controlled.

- Maximum total daily dose of 2 grams with concomitant liver disease or chronic alcohol consumption.

- Counsel patient not to exceed the recommended daily dose and to be especially aware if using other non-prescription and prescription products that may contain acetaminophen.

b. Non-steroidal anti-inflammatory drugs

  i. Recommended for patients who fail acetaminophen therapy or have inflammation.[2]

- All NSAIDs have relatively equal efficacy, but individual patient response differs among agents.

- Adequate trial duration of 2–3 weeks is necessary to assess efficacy.

- If trial of first agent fails, recommend trial of another NSAID until an effective agent for the patient is found.

- For patients with one or more of the following risk factors for gastrointestinal bleeding:

  - Age >65
  - Oral glucocorticoid use
  - History of peptic ulcer disease
  - History of upper GI bleed
  - Oral anticoagulant use
  - Co-morbid medical conditions

  One of the following regimens should be selected to reduce the risk of gastrointestinal injury:

  - NSAID + Proton-pump Inhibitor (PPI)

    Most commonly used and preferred regimen.

  - NSAID + misoprostol

    Not as well tolerated due to side effects, particularly diarrhea and flatulence, which occur in a dose-dependent manner.[3]

  - COX 2 selective NSAID (e.g., celecoxib)

    Due to the recent debate regarding increased cardiovascular risk in some patients with COX-2 selective NSAIDs, celecoxib is not recommended as a first-line agent. As with all medications, both risks and benefits must be discussed with the patient and his or her provider prior to initiation of therapy.

3. Options for patients who experience no relief from acetaminophen, capsaicin, and/or NSAIDs

    a. Intra-articular injections

        i. Glucocorticoid and hyaluronate injections are useful for the local treatment of knee pain and inflammation for patients who have not responded or have a contraindication to initial therapy with acetaminophen, NSAIDs, or non-pharmacologic measures.

    b. Glucosamine and chondroitin

        i. Patients may need to continue treatment for 1–3 months before seeing an effect; discontinue if no improvement after 3 months.[2]

        ii. Educate patients that the FDA does not adequately regulate these products because they are marketed as dietary supplements.

    c. Tramadol

        i. May be considered for patients with contraindications to NSAIDs, including impaired renal function, or in patients who have not responded to previous oral therapy.[3]

    d. Narcotics

        i. Patients who do not respond to or cannot tolerate any of the other agents mentioned thus far, who are actively participating in non-pharmacologic methods, and who continue to have severe pain, may be considered candidates for opioid therapy.[3] Low-dose narcotics are typically used (e.g., hydrocodone, codeine), usually given in combination with acetaminophen.[2]

    e. Surgery

        i. If pain is intolerable despite adequate trials of pharmacologic and non-pharmacologic treatment options, and if pain is limiting activities of daily living, joint replacement may be considered as an alternative to chronic narcotic use.[2]

Risk Assessment (Monitoring and Adverse Effects)

1. Acetaminophen

    a. Despite being one of the safest analgesics, acetaminophen still has its risks, predominantly hepatic toxicity. Use with caution in patients with liver disease. Avoid use in patients with chronic alcohol abuse.

2. NSAIDs

    a. In addition to the known risk of gastrointestinal injury and renal toxicity, recent data has shown that NSAIDs, particularly COX-2 selective NSAIDs, may increase the risk of thrombotic cardiovascular events, such as myocardial infarction or stroke.[3] As with all medications, both the provider and patient should discuss and weigh the potential risks and benefits of treatment with NSAIDs.

Patients at high risk include:

i. A history of peptic ulcer or GI bleed

ii. Renal insufficiency [characterized by increased serum creatinine (SCr) and BUN]

iii. Age >65

iv. Congestive heart failure or other cardiovascular risk. NSAIDs should not be used immediately before or after coronary artery bypass graft (CABG).[6]

v. Diuretic therapy

vi. Severe hepatic disease

Monitor for:

i. Elevated blood pressure

ii. Hyperkalemia

iii. Peripheral edema

While all patients taking NSAIDs should be monitored for the above-mentioned parameters, those who are deemed to be high risk should be monitored more closely.

Goals of Therapy

1. Relieve pain and minimize or prevent associated symptoms.
2. Improve and maintain functional joint mobility.
3. Improve or maintain quality of life.
4. Slow progression of the disease.
5. Avoid or minimize toxic effects of therapy.

Clinical Pharmacy Goals

1. Identify patients with pain secondary to osteoarthritis and ensure treatment with appropriate agents and doses.
2. Educate patients, caregivers, and family about OA and the prevention of disease progression.
3. Monitor patients for side effects of treatment.
4. Monitor and encourage adherence to treatment.
5. Increase patient awareness and use of non-pharmacologic treatment methods.

Outcome Measures

1. Process measures: Achieve symptom control, as evaluated by a decreased pain scale score, in a cost-effective manner; maintain and improve joint mobility.

2. Health outcome measures: Maintain and improve quality of life.

Patient Information Resources

1. http://www.arthritis.org

2. http://www.rheumatology.org

3. http://www.niams.nih.gov

4. http://www.aboutjoints.com/patientinfo/topics/osteoarthritis/Osteo-arthritis2.html

5. http://www.nhlbi.nih.gov/health/public/heart/obesity/wecan/learn-it/bmi-chart.htm

6. http://www.arthritis.org/events/getinvolved/ProgramsServices/ArthritisSelfHelp.asp

CASE STUDY

S: BK is a 185 pound, 5"4' 62-year-old female previously diagnosed with osteoarthritis of the knee. Acetaminophen 1 gram four times daily was started 5 weeks ago. After initiation of medication therapy, she noticed some improvement in her joint pain, but she states she still does not have complete relief of her symptoms. In fact, she reports that her symptoms sometimes feel worse. What are the next steps for treating BK's OA?

Allergies: NKA

Current medications:

Acetaminophen 1000 mg QID

Atenolol 25 mg once daily

Multivitamin once daily

O: BP 118/72, HR 70

BMI 31.8

A/P: Patient with OA with incomplete relief of symptoms.

1. A topical agent such as capsaicin may be warranted. *The addition of a topical agent such as capsaicin cream to acetaminophen therapy may provide additional pain relief. For best results, capsaicin cream should be applied three to four times a day on a regular basis. BK should be counseled to wash her hands well after each application, and be told that a local burning sensation at the site of application is common. If the patient can't tolerate the local side effects of capsaicin (e.g., burning/irritation sensation, redness, warmth),*

another topical option is a methylsalicylate cream (e.g., Ben-Gay cream), which may be applied as needed for pain.

2. Switch from acetaminophen to an NSAID if symptoms persist after adding capsaicin. *Failure of acetaminophen treatment warrants a trial with an NSAID. All NSAIDs are approximately equal in efficacy, although individual patient response will differ. Though BK does not have a history of peptic ulcer disease or GI bleeding, a non-acetylated salicylate should be considered first (e.g., salsalate, sodium salicylate, choline salicylate, magnesium salicylate) since they appear as effective as the other traditional NSAIDs with fewer GI side effects. If the first agent fails (after a trial of at least 2–3 weeks), another NSAID should be tried. In many cases, it is possible to use lower dosages of the NSAIDs to control the pain or only use the agent intermittently. Whichever therapy is chosen, the need for continuation of the treatment requires ongoing reassessment.*

3. Recommend and encourage the patient to enroll in a weight loss program. *BK is obese based on her BMI of 31.8. Her ideal or goal body weight for her height is between 110 and 140 pounds.[7] Since maintaining an appropriate body weight can be one of the most important factors in preventing osteoarthritis, losing weight may lead to improvement in her symptoms and joint mobility. Consider referral to a nutritionist and/or physical therapist at subsequent visits.*

4. Educate and counsel patient regarding the use of other self-management techniques. *In addition to weight loss, BK should be assessed for her understanding and use of other self-management techniques. Since non-pharmacologic methods are increasingly being recognized as an important part of effective OA management, patients should be educated on the various modalities currently available (e.g., physical therapy range-of-motion exercises, muscle-strengthening exercises, joint protection and rest, properly cushioned shoes).*

5. Follow-up with PCP in 4 weeks. *At subsequent visits, the patient should be assessed for adequate pain relief and medication side effects. The patient should be weighed, aiming for no more than a 1–2 pound weight loss per week. Discuss ongoing self-management techniques and help the patient set realistic goals. Encourage continued adherence to both non-pharmacologic and pharmacologic treatments.*

References

1.   National Institute of Arthritis and Musculoskeletal and Skin Diseases. Arthritis Prevalence Rising as Baby Boomers Grow Older: Osteoarthritis Second Only to Chronic Heart Disease in Worksite Disability. Available at http://www.niams.nih.gov/ ne/press/1998/05_05.htm. Accessed November 27, 2006.

2.   Hansen KE, Elliott ME. Osteoarthritis. In: Dipiro JT, Talbert RL, Yee GC, et al., eds. *Pharmacotherapy: a pathophysiologic approach.* 6th ed. New York, NY: The McGraw-Hill Companies, Inc; 2005:1685–1703.

3.   American College of Rheumatology Subcommittee on Osteoarthritis Guidelines. Recommendations for the medical management of osteoarthritis of the hip and knee. *Arthritis Rheum.* 2000; 43:1905–15. Available at http://www.rheumatology.org/ publications/guidelines/oa-mgmt/oa-mgmt.asp?aud=mem. Accessed April 14, 2006.

4.   Hinton R, Moody RL, Thomas SF. Osteoarthritis: Diagnosis and Therapeutic Considerations. *Am Fam Physician.* 2002; 65(5):841–8.

5.   Arthritis Foundation. Arthritis Foundation Self-Help Program. Available at http:// www.arthritis.org/events/getinvolved/ProgramsServices/ArthritisSelfHelp.asp Accessed November 2, 2006.

6.   Food and Drug Administration. Medication Guide for Non-Steroidal Anti-Inflammatory Drugs (NSAIDs). Available at www.fda.gov/cder/drug/infopage/ COX2/NSAIDmedguide.htm. Accessed November 8, 2006.

7.   National Heart, Lung, and Blood Institute. Standard BMI Calculator. Available at http://www.nhlbisupport.com/bmi/bmicalc.htm. Accessed October 11, 2006.

Major Depression

Tiffany Erickson

Depression affects an estimated 121 million people worldwide and is a leading cause of disability.[1] While depression can be reliably diagnosed and treated, it is often undiagnosed and undertreated, leading to a loss of productivity, functional decline, and increased mortality. Recognizing the need for improved management of depression, pharmacists play an important role in helping both providers and patients achieve treatment goals.

Depression often accompanies other chronic illnesses, including diabetes and cardiovascular disease, and its presence may predispose these patients to poorer outcomes. Furthermore, it is often difficult to manage other chronic illnesses if depression is uncontrolled because patients may lack capacity or motivation to adhere to medications and lifestyle recommendations. As a care provider, it is important for the pharmacist to consider the management of depression before advancing the treatment of other medical issues.

Indications

The management of depression is multi-faceted and best performed by providers with whom the patient has a trusting relationship. The depressed patient is typically followed most closely by his or her primary care provider (PCP) and other mental health specialists. However, due to the frequent monitoring and titration of medications needed, pharmacists play a significant role in collaborating on therapy management.

At our institution, the clinical pharmacist is most often involved in optimizing medication use once antidepressants have been prescribed. Examples of services provided include giving detailed and personal education on medications and depression, coordinating medication organizers to increase compliance with multiple medications, monitoring safety and other parameters by scheduling regular (weekly or biweekly) medication refills or phone calls, monitoring adherence by examining refill records, and consulting with the PCP when a patient's status changes.

Additional roles for the pharmacist who is experienced in working with depression include screening and management. Because the pharmacist is involved in ongoing management of other chronic conditions and is often the most accessible care provider, screening for depression could conveniently be done by the pharmacist. Depression should be suspected when patients have multiple unscheduled medical visits; frequent symptoms (e.g., unexplained somatic complaints, fatigue, irritability, sleep disturbances, appetite changes, and/or weight changes); work or relationship problems; or chronic impairing medical conditions (e.g., cancer or post-traumatic stress disorder). If these problems are identified, a depression screen should be considered. Multiple screening tools are available, but generally asking the following two questions is useful:[2]

- During the past month, have you often been bothered by feeling down, depressed, or hopeless?

- During the past month, have you often been bothered by having little interest or pleasure in doing things?

If the patient answers yes to either question, proceed with a follow-up interview to determine symptoms. See **Table 18-1** for the diagnostic criteria for symptoms.[3] If screening is positive, discuss findings with the patient's PCP.

Table 18-1. Criteria for Diagnosis of Major Depressive Episode[3]

Symptom	DSM-IV Diagnostic Criteria for Major Depressive Episode
Depressed mood*	Depressed mood most of the day, nearly every day, for at least 2 weeks
Anhedonia*	Markedly diminished interest or pleasure in almost all activities, for at least 2 weeks
Weight change	Substantial (5% or more change in 1 month) and unintentional weight loss or gain
Sleep disturbance	Insomnia or hypersomnia nearly every day
Psychomotor problems	Psychomotor agitation or retardation nearly every day
Lack of energy	Fatigue or loss of energy nearly every day
Excessive guilt	Feelings of worthlessness or excessive guilt nearly every day
Poor concentration	Diminished ability to think or concentrate nearly every day
Suicidal ideation	Recurrent thoughts of death or suicide

* At least one of these symptoms must be present, along with three to four or more of the additional symptoms (need five positive symptoms total).

Patients who have a diagnosis of depression and need pharmacotherapy can be referred to a pharmacist for ongoing medication management.

Management

Once a diagnosis of depression is considered, rule out and treat causes of secondary depression, including other medical illnesses, medication side effects (including withdrawal effects), and substance abuse. If they are addressed and depression still exists, proceed to pharmacotherapy as indicated.

Before initiating therapy, determine illness severity (mild, moderate, or severe) depending on the degree of functional impairment. Mild depression may be watched or treated with non-pharmacologic options such as psychotherapy. Moderate to severe depression warrants an antidepressant trial as initial therapy.

The majority of depressed patients have a response to at least one antidepressant; however, individual agents are effective in only 50–60% of patients.[2] Therefore, it may be time consuming and require several medication trials to find the most effective regimen for any given patient. Due to the comparable efficacy between and within classes of antidepressant medications, initial selection is based on previous personal or first-degree relative use of an antidepressant, anticipated side effects and safety concerns, potential drug–drug and drug–disease interactions, patient preference, convenience (e.g., pharmacokinetic parameters), and financial considerations.

Those with a personal or family history of use will often respond similarly. Without prior use information, it is very difficult to predetermine patient response to an antidepressant, both between and within drug classes, because variability exists among individuals. Clinical trials show little differences in tolerability or efficacy among antidepressants.[4] For example, while some patients experience sedation on a given antidepressant, other patients will experience insomnia. When patients *do* find success with a particular agent, they may continue it indefinitely. For this reason, in the absence of contraindications, it is more cost effective to start with a generic antidepressant and monitor response. Some medications may also be more effective when concurrent conditions are present. See **Table 18-2** for a guide to choosing initial pharmacotherapy based on select patient characteristics.

When starting a medication, begin with a low dose and titrate up slowly as side effects permit. For elderly patients and those with underlying anxiety disorders or suspected bipolar disorder, start at half the recommended initiation dose.

After initiating antidepressant pharmacotherapy, the pharmacist's education and counseling is critical. Many patients stop their medications before an adequate trial is complete due to the lack of immediate effects or initial side effects. Proper counseling helps to minimize incomplete drug trials and provides the patient with more options for medication management. Family members

Table 18-2. Guide to Choosing Initial Therapy Based on Selected Patient Characteristics

Medication Class	Medication	Preferred in	Avoid/Use Caution in
Selective serotonin reuptake inhibitor (SSRI)	Fluoxetine Fluvoxamine Paroxetine Citalopram Sertraline Escitalopram	Fluoxetine has a long half-life and therefore is a good choice for non-adherent patients Children and adolescents Elderly Risk for overdose Depression coinciding with panic, OCD, or psychomotor retardation Pregnancy	Insomnia Sexual dysfunction Renal dysfunction Bipolar disorder
Tricyclic antidepressant	Amitriptyline Nortriptyline Desipramine Maprotiline Imipramine Clomipramine	Depression with melancholic features or agitation Severe major depression Depression with: Insomnia Migraine Chronic pain Neuropathic pain	Benign prostatic hypertrophy, cardiovascular disease, elderly, dementia, glaucoma, renal dysfunction, suicidal ideation, risk for overuse, obesity, postural instability, seizure disorder, sexual dysfunction, drug interactions
Serotonin-norepinephrine reuptake inhibitor (SNRI)	Venlafaxine	Concurrent pain History of postural hypotension	History of stroke Hypertension Renal dysfunction Sexual dysfunction
	Duloxetine	Peripheral neuropathy Sexual dysfunction	
Norepinephrine-dopamine reuptake inhibitor (NDRI)	Bupropion	Smoking cessation, overweight, somnolence, GI side effects	Seizure disorder, anorexia/bulimia, head injury
Miscellaneous	Nefazodone	Sexual dysfunction, sleep disorders, postpartum depression, depression with anxiety	Elevated baseline LFTs, active liver disease, hepatotoxicity, alcoholism, concurrent drugs metabolized by CYP 3A4
	Mirtazipine	Insomnia, anxiety, weight loss, sexual dysfunction	Risk of agranulocytosis, myelosuppressive disorder, overweight
	Trazodone	Insomnia	Male gender (risk of priapism), postural hypotension
	St John's Wort	Patient preference, mild cases only (no evidence of efficacy over placebo)	Moderate or severe depression, drug interactions
Monoamine oxidase inhibitor (MAOI)	Selegiline	Refractory depression	

Adapted from references 2 and 5.

and/or caretakers should be included in the education sessions whenever possible. Counseling should emphasize the:

- Recognition that depression is a highly prevalent but treatable medical illness
- Pharmacotherapy indication and medication instructions
- Expected side effects and any special monitoring needed
- Reassurance that some side effects may diminish with continued adherence, especially if the depression improves
- Reassurance that it takes time for the beneficial effects to be noticed
- Possibility that the dose will be increased slowly over time, which may delay the time to therapeutic response
- Importance of the patient being accessible for follow-up as part of the treatment plan
- Need to continue the medication even after feeling better
- Need to consult with providers before discontinuing or lowering the dose of the medication
- Importance of obtaining timely refills; a review of prescription refill procedures may be needed
- Signs and symptoms of worsening or recurring depression
- Contact information for the pharmacist and PCP and what to do if problems arise
- Available information resources (see Patient Information Resources listed below)

After starting medication, prompt follow-up is needed. Because the physician may not have as much time to spend with a patient following pharmacotherapy initiation, pharmacists are often involved in providing initial follow-up, either via telephone or in clinic. Areas of evaluation include suicide risk, medication tolerability, and efficacy.

The most important aspect of initial follow-up is assessment of suicide risk. This should be done 1–2 weeks after starting medication, and periodically thereafter. This is accomplished through an assessment of the presence of suicidal or homicidal ideation, intent, or plans; access to means for suicide and the lethality of those means; presence of psychotic symptoms, command hallucinations, or severe anxiety; presence of alcohol or substance abuse; history and seriousness of previous attempts; and family history of or recent exposure to suicide. Unfortunately, predictability of this assessment is so poor that negative responses do not rule out suicide risk. If risk for suicide is present, immediately notify the PCP and other health care providers. It is prudent for the clinical pharmacist to work closely with social workers, case managers, and other mental health professionals.

Tolerability of medication and presence of side effects must also be assessed. This should be done 2–4 weeks after initiating pharmacotherapy to give an adequate trial. If side effects are present, consider the following options:

- Provide reassurance and watch and wait (assuming no immediate medical risk, and patient is agreeable and maintains compliance)

- Alter the medication dose, frequency, or time of administration

- Change to a different medication (within class is considered acceptable until two failures within the same class, or switch to a new class)

- Provide specific treatment for side effects

If manic symptoms (e.g., elevated mood, increased energy, impulsivity) emerge after starting therapy, this indicates the diagnosis may be bipolar disorder and the patient should be promptly referred to the PCP.

At least 4 weeks after the patient has been compliant on a stable dose of medication, an assessment of efficacy is needed. Review symptoms of depression listed in Table 18-1. At least a moderate improvement (>50%) in symptoms and functioning is expected, although the ultimate goal of therapy is elimination of symptoms. If partial (26–49% decrease in baseline severity of symptoms) or no response (<25% decrease in baseline severity of symptoms), assess how compliant the patient was with the medication and optimize adherence as indicated. Consider obtaining drug levels if warranted, such as when subjective information does not correspond with the clinical picture or refill history.

If the patient is compliant with current therapy and not responding as expected, notify the PCP who should consider revision of the treatment plan. Options include:

- Increasing the dose of antidepressant if patient has partial or no response. Reassess and continue titration if needed.

- Changing to another medication within the same class. Often a patient may fail one drug in a class but may respond to or tolerate another.

- Changing to a different class of antidepressants.

- If there is a partial response, consider augmenting with an additional agent such as a mood stabilizer, or combining antidepressants with different mechanisms.

- Considering alternative therapies, including non-pharmacologic therapies.

If an antidepressant is discontinued, the pharmacist may assist with management of cross-tapering as indicated.

If patient response is adequate to meet goals (>50% response), the regimen should be continued and the pharmacist may no longer be needed for monitoring. If there is no recurrence or relapse for at least 6–12 months from time of symptom remission, consider tapering off of pharmacotherapy. Slowly decrease dose over several weeks and monitor for withdrawal effects and the return of depressive symptoms, which would require resuming full-dose pharmacotherapy. If this is not the first episode of major depression or the patient has severe depression with a high risk of suicide, consider indefinite treatment with antidepressant medication.

Goals of Therapy

1. Achieve and sustain symptom remission.
2. Restore occupational and psychosocial functioning.
3. Decrease the likelihood of relapses and recurrence.

Clinical Pharmacy Goals

1. Screen patients for depression and facilitate follow-up with PCP.
2. Educate patients, family, and caregiver regarding depression as a treatable medical illness.
3. Recommend safe, well-tolerated, and cost-effective therapeutic regimens.
4. Maximize adherence to prescribed regimen, and monitor for overuse and noncompliance.
5. Minimize adverse outcomes of therapy, including withdrawal reactions (assist in refills/continuity of care).
6. Minimize and manage drug interactions and medication side effects.
7. Be accessible for follow-up, especially with pharmacotherapy initiation and dose escalations.
8. Monitor medication safety by evaluating suicide risk and collaborate with other health care professionals when risk is identified to assure medication is not taken more frequently than prescribed.
9. Assist with management of chemically or medically induced causes of depression (e.g., thyroid disorders, medication-associated, etc.).

Outcome Measures

1. Process measures: Change in depressive symptoms; time in remission; change in occupational and psychosocial functioning; rates of medication adherence; rates of adverse medication effects.
2. Health outcome measures: Number of unscheduled clinic visits; patient and family satisfaction.

Patient Information Resources

1. Treatment Works. Major Depressive Disorder, A Patient and Family Guide. Developed from the American Psychiatric Association Practice Guidelines: http://www.psych.org.

2. Screening for depression: recommendations from the U.S. Preventative Services Task Force. summaries for patients. *Ann Intern Med.* 2002; May 21:136(10):I56.

3. http://www.healthyminds.org/multimedia/depression.pdf

References

1. World Health Organization. Depression. Available at http://www.who.int/mental_health/management/depression/definition/en/. Accessed November 2006.

2. Whooley MA, Simon GE. Managing depression in medical outpatients. *N Engl J Med.* 2000; 343:1942–50.

3. American Psychiatric Association. *Diagnostic and statistical manual of mental disorders,* 4th ed. DSM-IV. Washington, DC: American Psychiatric Association; 1994.

4. Mann JJ. The medical management of depression. *N Engl J Med.* 2005; 353:1819–34.

5. Premera Blue Cross. Clinical Practice Guideline: Diagnosis and Treatment of Major Depression in Adults in the Primary Care Setting. Updated 2004. Available at https://www.premera.com/stellent/groups/public/documents/pdfs/dynwat%3B4308_4386672_3836.pdf. Accessed June 19, 2006.

Bibliography

1. American Psychiatric Association. *Treating major depressive disorder: a quick reference guide.* Based on *practice guideline for the treatment of patients with major depressive disorder,* 2nd ed. Arlington, VA: American Psychiatric Association; 2002.

2. Remick RA. Diagnosis and management of depression in primary care: a clinical update and review. *CMAJ.* 2002; 167:1253–60.

3. U.S. Preventative Services Task Force. Screening for depression: recommendations and rationale. *Ann Intern Med.* 2002; 136:760–4.

Travel Medicine

Tiffany Erickson

Travel medicine is the provision of health care for international travelers. An estimated 50 million people travel every year from industrialized nations to tropical or subtropical destinations, and up to 70% of these travelers report health problems while abroad.[1–5] Diarrhea is the most commonly reported morbidity, and the leading causes of mortality include cardiovascular disease, trauma, and infectious disease.[4] Many of the risks that international travelers are exposed to can be minimized by taking appropriate precautions. Providing education for international travelers on disease prevention and risk minimization is an important service provided by travel medicine specialists.

Travel medicine is often considered a specialized field with services provided by experts outside of the primary care setting. The population we serve in our institution includes a large number of immigrants who frequently return home to developing countries to visit friends and relatives (VFRs), usually for longer than 30 days. VFRs account for an estimated 40% of international travelers and have many barriers to care that are often not present for typical tourist or business travelers.[4–6] In order for these patients to have adequate access and culturally appropriate pre-travel planning, travel medicine is a service we provide in our primary care clinics. The service we provide is geared toward the unique population we serve, which may not be applicable to all types of travelers; our pharmacists are not specialists in travel medicine. This chapter is meant to serve as an introductory guide to providing travel medicine consults, especially for VFRs, and is not all-inclusive. However, many excellent online and print resources are referenced for your review.

Indications

Travel consults can be offered for anyone who is planning international travel. Those traveling exclusively to Canada, Australia, New Zealand, Japan, or Western Europe are considered low-risk for travel-related illness, and no specific travel-related medications or vaccinations are required. However, travelers to these areas may require coordination of care for chronic medical conditions and prescriptions, especially if the travel is for an extended period of time.

Due to the time and intensity involved with travel medicine coordination, our recommendation is that patients must have an appointment scheduled with the pharmacist specifically to address travel medicine. As with all our pharmacist-managed consultations, a referral from the primary care provider (PCP) must be documented in the patient's chart. Ideally, travelers should plan well in advance and appointments should be set at least 1 month before travel. Those with more urgent departures can be seen but may not get adequate preventative care, as it may take several weeks to assure completion of vaccination series and development of adequate immunity. Malaria prophylaxis may need to be started 1 week or more before departure, and the coordination of chronic medication refills, especially for patients with insurance plans, may require time to process.

It can take a considerable amount of time (more than 60 minutes) to coordinate and provide travel consultations, especially for travelers with incomplete medical records, no history of international travel, or multiple medical conditions. Additionally, patients may not retain all the information if given at once and some may need to return for assessment of labs/virology or for second immunizations. Therefore, we prefer to divide the pre-travel consult into two shorter visits if the itinerary allows.

Management

Pre-travel consultation should include at a minimum:

1. *Interview and/or chart review.* Obtain a detailed travel itinerary, including departure and return date or estimated length of stay, all anticipated destinations (including layovers), lodging (hotel, house, camp, etc.), reason for travel and anticipated activities. Accessibility to resources and ability to use and implement pre-travel medication and education appropriately should also be addressed.

   Obtain patient history, including prior travel history and any previous education received, prior travel-related illness or injury, immunization history, virology (if unsure of previous vaccination status) and other pertinent labs, childhood diseases or other exposure to communicable diseases, current medications, medical history, allergies, and financial constraints or insurance coverage.

2. *Use of travel information resources (refer to resources section).* Disease outbreaks may occur at any given destination at any time. Referring to a reliable, up-to-date source of outbreak and travel information is vital for ensuring that you are providing appropriate recommendations. Excellent online and print resources are available. Two sources we commonly use are www.cdc.gov/travel, which is free and updated frequently, and www.travax.com, by Shoreland, Inc, which is easy to navigate and updated regularly but *does* require an annual subscription. Other print sources are available (see references) and may be updated regularly.

3. *Risk assessment and provision of care.* Based on the above information, assess potential exposure risks and individual patient characteristics and consider:

   a. *Immunizations.* As part of travel consultation, the pharmacist should assess the need for both routine and travel-related immunizations. In some states, pharmacists may become certified to administer immunizations; however, these vaccines are commonly given in clinic by nursing or medical assistants.

      i. Routine immunizations. Routine immunizations that are not up-to-date should be completed as necessary and as time allows. Diseases that are no longer endemic in the United States may still pose risks to the international traveler. A consultation for travel is an excellent time for the pharmacist to review and update routine immunizations. These include tetanus, diphtheria, pertussis, varicella, measles, mumps, rubella, *haemophilus influenza* type b, influenza, pneumococcal, and polio. Hepatitis A, hepatitis B, and meningococcal are also indicated for children and some adults, although many adults may not have had these as routine immunizations. Some vaccines may be given on an accelerated schedule to allow for completion before upcoming travel. Review references for specifics of vaccine administration, timing, and contraindications.

      ii. Travel-related immunizations. In addition to the above routine immunizations, recommend immunizations for travel according to destination. Vaccinations available in the United States to consider for travel include the following:

         • Hepatitis A. Hepatitis A transmission occurs via contaminated food and water as the result of poor hygiene or sanitation. The virus can be inactivated with heat, therefore cooking food thoroughly and boiling water are excellent ways to prevent transmission. Hepatitis A vaccine is an inactivated vaccine and is given as two doses, 6 months apart. Some protection can be obtained without the primary series for a traveler who is leaving in less than 6 months. After one dose of vaccine, protective antibody levels are achieved in 88% of patients in 15 days and 95–99% after 30 days.[1,7] Hepatitis A immune globulin can be considered for unvaccinated travelers leaving for endemic areas in <15 days or at-risk infants <1 year old.

- Hepatitis B. Hepatitis B is transmitted through contact with infected body fluids or contaminated blood products, which are often a concern in the developing world. Hepatitis B vaccine is given in a three-injection series at 0, 1, and 6 months; no boosters are recommended. Counseling on protected intercourse and avoidance of contaminated blood (via dental work, tattooing, acupuncture, and other medical procedures, for example) may minimize chance of exposure.

  Those with previous exposure to hepatitis A or B will have lifetime immunity and this can be determined by checking antibody titers. Because the majority of our traveling patients are immigrants from hepatitis endemic areas and have undocumented exposure to hepatitis or vaccination status, we find checking for hepatitis A and B antibodies is a very cost-effective way to determine who needs the vaccination series.

- Typhoid. Typhoid fever is a common cause of acute febrile illness in the international traveler and can be life threatening. Travelers contract the bacteria through ingestion of contaminated foods and beverages. Typhoid vaccinations protect against *Salmonella typhi* but do not protect against other strains of *salmonella*; both strains can cause typhoid fever. Therefore, education on food and water precautions is an important way to prevent contamination, as is vaccination. Typhoid vaccine should be completed at least 14 days prior to exposure for optimal protection against *Salmonella typhi*. Typhoid vaccination is contraindicated in children <2 years old. There are two typhoid vaccinations available in the United States:

  - Oral typhoid vaccine (OTV) is a live attenuated strain of *Salmonella typhi*, strain Ty21a. The capsules are taken every other day for a total of four doses. Because OTV is inactivated by heat, it must be refrigerated and taken with cool liquids. Efficacy rates are 43–96% in protecting against typhoid.[7] Contraindications include immunosuppression, pregnancy, and abnormal gastrointestinal function. Concurrent use of antibiotics, including some anti-malarials, may lessen the vaccine's efficacy, and is not recommended. Boosters are recommended at 5-year intervals when using oral typhoid; therefore, OTV is a good option for those who travel to risk areas frequently.

- Typhoid Vi capsular polysaccharide (CPS) vaccine is injectable, given as one dose. It has protective efficacy rates ranging 60–95%.[7] Because it is an inactivated vaccine, it has fewer contraindications and interactions with antibiotics. CPS is a good option for patients with compliance issues, who are leaving shortly, or who don't have refrigeration. The duration of immunity is less than with OTV; boosters are recommended at 2-year intervals when injectable typhoid is administered.

• Meningococcal. Meningococcal disease occurs primarily in sub-Saharan Africa during the months December through June, and where individuals are living in close quarters, such as a college dormitory. It is *recommended* that travelers with exposure risks are offered meningococcal vaccine. Currently, meningococcal vaccine is *required* for travelers going to Saudi Arabia to make pilgrimage to Mecca, as epidemics of meningococcal disease have occurred in this setting. Meningococcal vaccine is given as a single dose. There are currently two meningococcal vaccinations available:

- Meningococcal polysaccharide vaccine (Menomune™) is licensed for patients over 2 years of age. Boosters are recommended at 3–5 year intervals.

- Meningococcal quadrivalent conjugate vaccine (Menactra™) is indicated for those aged 11–55 years and may confer longer immunity than Menomune™. Booster interval has not yet been determined. Case reports of Guillain-Barré syndrome in patients who received Menactra™ are currently being investigated and patients need to be counseled on this risk.

• Yellow fever. Documentation of yellow fever vaccination, or letter of exemption based on contraindications, is an entry requirement for certain destinations, and is recommended for many travelers. Yellow fever is a live, attenuated viral vaccine that has very specific storage and reconstitution requirements and only centers that are certified to meet the requirements are authorized to administer it. The vaccine is protective 10 days after administration, and a booster is recommended every 10 years. Contraindications include egg allergy, pregnancy, lactation, compromised immunity, and patients <9 months old. Although extremely rare, there have been cases of serious neurologic and viscerotropic diseases reported in travelers who have received the vaccine, especially in those >60 years. Risks and benefits should be discussed.

- Polio. Polio still circulates in some developing countries and should be considered for travelers to endemic areas. The primary series for unvaccinated adults is three doses, given at 0, 1, and 6 months. Adults that have had primary vaccination with polio will need a booster before travel to endemic areas.

- Influenza. Travelers are at high risk for respiratory infections, including influenza. Exposure depends on destination and the time of year. Transmission occurs year-round in the tropics. Travelers going to endemic areas should get a vaccine prior to departure if they have not already received it for the current season. Influenza vaccine does not provide protection against avian influenza.

- Rabies. Rabies is transmitted via a bite or scratch from an infected animal and is almost always fatal if not properly treated. Those planning adventure hiking, backpacking, camping, visiting family farm, or other outdoor activities with exposure to animals are at risk. Vaccination eliminates the need for rabies immune globulin, which can be difficult to obtain in the developing world. Those with risk and without timely access to postexposure prophylaxis are candidates for the rabies vaccine. The vaccine is given as three injections: at 0, 1, and 3–4 weeks. Boosters can be considered every 2–3 years depending on exposure. Education regarding discouraging travelers, especially children, from touching local animals while abroad is important. If contact occurs, it is critical to seek immediate care for bites or scratches.

- Japanese encephalitis (JE). JE is an emerging infection, transmitted to humans by *Culex* mosquitoes with pigs as the reservoir. Therefore, those planning an extended trip in certain rural farming areas are at greatest risk for infection. JE is an inactivated vaccine. Three injections, at least 1 week apart, are needed for optimal protection, although two doses may confer up to 80% protection. Boosters are recommended every 3 years if exposure is repeated. There is a low but severe risk of hypersensitivity reactions to JE vaccine. Patients should be observed for 30 minutes after administration and advised not to travel for at least 10 days after the last dose as there is a risk of delayed hypersensitivity.

iii. For any vaccines recommended, counsel on indication, potential side effects, and recommended follow-up for completion of series. Provide patient with Vaccine Information Statement. Document any recommended vaccines given or declined in patient's medical chart and record on patient immunization record to give to patients. Provide contact information for clinics that can provide recommended/required immunizations not offered by your institution. Our institution does not carry yellow fever and rabies vaccines, so patients are referred to the Public Health Department or other sites for these immunizations if needed.

If vaccine status is undocumented and patient cannot confirm previous exposure, it is usually better to err on the side of caution and give the vaccine. If there is not time to complete an indicated vaccination series, giving as many doses as possible (without exceeding recommended intervals) may confer some benefit and is recommended.

b. *Malaria chemoprophylaxis.* Malaria is a very common but preventable cause of illness in travelers going to tropical destinations.[8,9] It is the most common cause of death due to infection in travelers.[10] Malaria chemoprophylaxis is effective when taken appropriately. Since risk of acquiring malaria and drug resistance patterns differ widely depending on specific destinations, consult a travel reference for recommendations on prophylaxis. Note that elevation and proximity to water may alter the risk area-to-area within a country, so obtaining a very specific itinerary is helpful. The maps at www.travax.com illustrate this best and are a good tool for patients to identify destinations.

Available malaria chemoprophylaxis regimens are listed in **Table 19-1**. The choice of an antimalarial agent should be based on resistance patterns at destination, contraindications, interactions, side effects anticipated, patient preference for dosing regimen, and cost considerations. Patients should be counseled on when to take the drug, how to manage side effects, and how to recognize the symptoms of malaria, which may present even after leaving endemic areas. Instructions on when to take the drug need to be very specific, especially if the patient is traveling on an extended trip to different areas with different risks. They may not need prophylaxis during their entire trip, but only before, during, and after travel to risk areas. Our institution cares for many patients with minimal or no prescription insurance. Travel medicine is considered elective and is not a covered service under our indigent care program. As previously mentioned, our patients often travel for longer than 30 days. Therefore, we most often use doxycycline as the anti-malarial of choice as it is the least expensive agent and is equally effective in most areas. In some cases, prescriptions for self-treatment of a malarial outbreak may be considered, especially in the long-term traveler.[11]

Counseling on avoidance of mosquito bites is also an effective way to prevent malaria. Mosquitoes that transmit malaria bite at night; therefore, minimizing outdoor exposure from dusk to dawn can help prevent

Table 19-1. Malaria Chemoprophylaxis Regimens

Drug	Efficacy[1]	Adult Dose	Pediatric Dose[2]	Common or Severe Side Effects	Contraindications/ Precautions	Approximate Cost per Tab[4]
Atovaquone/ Proguanil (Malarone)	98–100%	250 mg daily, start 1 day before exposure, continue x 7 days after.	5–8 kg: ½ pediatric tablet[3] 9–10 kg: ¾ pediatric tablet 11–20 kg: 1 pediatric tablet or ¼ adult tablet 21–30 kg: 2 pediatric tablets or ½ adult tablet 31–40 kg: 3 pediatric tablets or ¾ adult tablet > 40 kg: adult dose	Headaches, GI upset	Active liver or kidney disease	$6.00
Chloroquine phosphate (Aralen)	Not reported High rates of resistance in certain areas.	500 mg weekly, start 1 week before exposure and continue x 4 weeks after	8.3 mg/kg, maximum 500 mg	GI upset Transient blurred vision	Active kidney or liver disease Epilepsy Psoriasis	$5.00
Doxycycline (generics)	96.3%–99%	100 mg daily, start 1 day before exposure, continue x 4 weeks after	1.5–2 mg/kg, maximum 100 mg	Photosensitivity Vaginal candidiasis GI upset	Children <8 years old Do not administer with calcium or iron simultaneously	$0.30

Table 19-1. Malaria Chemoprophylaxis Regimens [cont'd]

Mefloquine (Lariam)	98%	5 mg./kg. to the nearest quarter tablet[5]	Common: Dizziness, GI upset, headaches, sleep disturbances, mood changes. Severe but less common: Neuropsychiatric changes (hallucinations, depression, visual disturbances) and seizures.	Psychiatric illness Cardiac arrhythmias Seizure disorder	$10.00
		250 mg weekly, start at least 1 week before exposure and continue x 4 weeks after (Consider starting 3–4 weeks before to monitor for psychiatric effects)			
Primaquine phosphate[6]	75–94%	0.8 mg/kg, maximum 52.6 mg	GI upset Hemolytic anemia in G6PD deficient patients	G6PD level mandatory before use	$1.00
		52.6 mg (2 tabs) daily, start 1 day before exposure, continue x 7 days after			

1 Based on efficacy rates at preventing malaria (parasitemia) by *P. falciparum* vs. placebo in controlled clinical trials. Data from Micromedex®.

2 Dosing frequency same as for adult.

3 Pediatric tablet is 62.5 mg atovaquone/25 mg proguanil per tablet.

4 Based on outpatient cost according to drugstore.com and walgreens.com.

5 Available as 250 mg tablets.

6 Malaria prophylaxis is off label use.

the disease. However, daytime insect precautions are also important for avoidance of diseases such as dengue, which are carried by day-biting mosquitoes. Patients should be counseled on using mosquito repellant containing meta-N,N-diethyl toluamide (DEET) 30–35%, staying in air conditioned rooms if possible, and using netting and protective clothing impregnated with insecticide. Picaridin may be as effective as DEET, but in the United States it is available in a much lower strength than was used to show efficacy in clinical trials, so it should not be recommended in place of DEET.

c. *Traveler's diarrhea (TD)*. TD is the most common cause of morbidity in travelers. Approximately 10–60% of travelers report having diarrhea while abroad.[1–3] In the majority of cases, a bacterial pathogen is identified, indicating the need for antibiotic treatment. Viral and parasitic causes are also identified but much less often and are usually seen in the long-term traveler. Education on food and water precautions can minimize risks of acquiring infectious diarrhea.

Self-treatment regimens for TD are listed in **Table 19-2**. Self-treatment should be limited to patients who understand the indication; it does not replace the need to seek care for severe diarrhea. Our institution does not routinely offer prescriptions for traveler's diarrhea self-treatment. This decision was based on post-travel follow-up data that revealed a large percentage of patients used the medication inappropriately for other illnesses, took it before departure, or gave it away to family members or friends during travel.[12] Instead, we focus on providing education. This should cover the importance of clean food and water, proper hygiene, fluid replacement, use of oral rehydration solutions, identifying signs and symptoms of dysentery (diarrhea associated with fevers, blood, mucus, cramping, nausea, or lasting longer than 48 hours), and when to seek care.

Table 19-2. Regimens for Self-Treatment of Traveler's Diarrhea

Drug	Dose	Comments
Ciprofloxacin	500 mg bid x 3 days	Not for use in children <18 years old
Levofloxacin	500 mg daily x 3 days	Not for use in children <18 years old
Azithromycin	500 mg x 1, then 250 mg daily x 4 days, or 1000 mg once	For areas with fluoroquinolone resistance
Loperamide	4 mg x 1, then 2 mg after each loose stool, no more than 16 mg in 24 hours	Use only in mild to moderate diarrhea with no evidence of dysentery
Rifaximin	200 mg tid x 3 days	Only for diarrhea presumed due to *E. coli* (no evidence of dysentery) Only indicated for those aged 12–65 years

d. *Education*. It is necessary to provide travel health advice for the prevention of disease or injury. Because of the time involved in providing individualized education, the physician is not always able to provide in-depth education, especially in the primary care setting. Therefore, referral to a pharmacist is an excellent opportunity for the patient to get the education needed. The pharmacists at our institution can provide immunizations or travel medications under prescriptive authority, but sometimes patients will have this done by their PCP and the pharmacist consult will be predominantly for travel education. Use travel references to find up-to-date recommendations for individual destinations and considerations for appropriate education; details on what the education should entail are also included.

Education can include, but is not limited to, discussion of the following topics:

i. Food and water precautions

ii. Prevention and self-management of diarrhea

iii. Use of sunscreen (especially with photosensitizing medications)

iv. Use of insect repellant, netting, and other avoidance measures

v. Sexually transmitted diseases (STDs) and blood-borne illness precautions

vi. Traffic and pedestrian safety

vii. Personal safety measures and avoidance of crime

viii. Deep venous thrombosis (DVT) prevention

ix. Considerations for travel insurance

x. Avoidance of freshwater swimming and walking barefoot

xi. Altitude sickness

xii. Avoidance of contact with animals

xiii. Local outbreaks of disease and protective measures

xiv. When to seek medical help

Additionally, as applicable, provide education on disease state management that may be affected by travel (e.g. insulin storage, fluctuating blood sugars, DVT risk, respiratory disease, dehydration, etc.). For those who will be in flight >7 hours, providing compression stockings has been shown to decrease rates of DVT and is a simple, well-tolerated treatment.[13] The patient information resources listed in a later section provide printed education for many of the topics above.

It is important to note that some patients, including many we care for at our institution, are unable to implement education given due to inaccessibility, financial barriers, cultural beliefs, or misunderstanding. Travelers to remote, rural areas also may not have the ability to implement education. For instance, things like hand soap, seat belts, flushing toilets, and refrigeration are not always accessible. Cultural or religious beliefs may discourage the use of protection during intercourse, and condoms obtained abroad may be poor quality. VFRs may not understand the need to take precautions when returning home to their native country. They may have had immune protection against illnesses such as malaria and typhoid, but that immunity can be lost when they come to the developed world for a period of time. They may not understand the importance of disease prevention when returning to their home, and this may make convincing them to pay for travel-related medications difficult. Even if VFRs have adequate resources and understanding, they may find it offensive to eat or act differently than their friends and family and will not feel comfortable following food, beverage, or other precautions. While it is important to give appropriate education, providing protection to these patients via vaccination and medication ahead of time is very helpful in preventing disease transmission.

e. *Medication coordination.* Ensure that the patient will have enough medication for managing chronic conditions for the duration of travel. If the medication supply needed is not covered on the patient's insurance plan due to larger quantities needed, the patient may need to work with his or her insurance company to get an authorization, or should be encouraged to pay out-of-pocket as a part of the trip expense so medication therapy is not interrupted. It may be possible to withhold some less vital medications (e.g., vitamins, pain relievers) or switch to a less expensive but therapeutically similar agent during travel. If the latter is done, it should be started well before travel to assess efficacy and tolerability.

f. *Special populations.* There are many populations of travelers that require special considerations for provision of travel medicine. These include infants, pregnant or lactating women, immunocompromised patients, health care workers, and the elderly. Risks and benefits of providing individual vaccinations and medications need to be weighed. Education should also be individualized. Consult references provided for more detailed information.

4. *Travel follow-up.* A post-travel visit should be considered, especially if the travel consultation occurs within the primary care clinic or outcomes are being tracked. Alternatively, patients can be advised on when and where to seek care if any concerns arise after travel.

During the post-travel visit, outcomes related to travel including worsening of existing chronic diseases should be evaluated. Any potential travel-related illnesses should promptly be reported to the patient's PCP for further assessment. Other travel follow-up by the pharmacist should include an assessment of how the patient utilized pre-travel education as well as how the patient tolerated and complied with travel medications. The pharmacist can assist with coordinating the patient's return visit to the PCP or other providers and supply any medication refills needed in the interim, if they provide refill authorization services.

The post-travel visit should also include completion of any vaccination series initiated prior to travel, as needed. If there is not documentation of a positive PPD test prior to travel and the traveler was at risk for contracting tuberculosis, a PPD skin test should be done after travel. Those at highest risk include travelers to endemic areas, especially for more than 30 days, or health care workers providing care abroad. The skin test should be placed 12 weeks after return to allow time for seroconversion should the patient have been exposed. Additionally, consider treatment of parasites if indicated, depending on destination and dietary habits during travel. Albendazole 400 mg daily for 5 days as presumptive treatment has been shown to be cost effective in the treatment of intestinal parasites, and it can be prescribed in the absence of contraindications.[14]

Our institution is a member of GeoSentinel, the global surveillance network that tracks and reports data on travel-related outcomes. To help the network detect and assess trends on travel-related morbidity, we are required to report any illnesses seen in the returned traveler. Any clinic that provides regular travel consultations should consider becoming a member of this important monitoring network. More information can be found at www.istm.org/geosentinel/main.html.

Goals of Therapy

1. To provide individualized, cost-effective, preventative health care for patients planning travel abroad.

2. To minimize risk of adverse travel-related outcomes including illness, injury, and medication-related side effects.

Clinical Pharmacy Goals

1. Conduct a patient interview and review medical records to obtain pertinent history.

2. Assess the individual's risks and patient-specific factors, to provide appropriate malaria prophylaxis, immunizations, traveler's diarrhea self-treatment, education, and coordination of medical care and prescriptions.

3. Facilitate getting routine immunization schedule up to date.

4. Educate on risks related to travel and measures to prevent illness or injury.

5. Document vaccines administered, travel-related medications recommended and prescribed, and education given.

6. Provide follow-up after completion of travel, including documentation of any adverse events and completion of applicable vaccination series.

7. Assess utility of pre-travel counseling to perform quality assurance and modify practice as needed.

Outcome Measures

1. Process measures: Compliance with prescription medication and travel recommendations; adverse events from travel-related medication and vaccinations; accessibility of documentation.

2. Health outcome measures: Travel-related illness and injury; health care utilization; patient and provider satisfaction.

Resources

For more information on setting up a travel medicine clinic or service, see www.travax.com under the section on Clinic Operations, and the book, *Travel Medicine*, both of which have information on the administrative procedures for setting up a travel medicine clinic. These resources include advice on recommended supplies and equipment, forms, policies and procedures, marketing, and more.

Patient Information Resources

1. Centers for Disease Control and Prevention: http://www.cdc.gov/travel

2. Shoreland, Inc.: http://www.tripprep.com

Provider Resources

Clinical Practice Guideline
Hill DR, Ericsson CD, Pearson RD, et al. The practice of travel medicine: guidelines by the Infectious Diseases Society of America. *Clin Infect Dis.* 2006; 43:1499–539.

Websites
1. American Society of Tropical Medicine and Hygiene: http://www.astmh.org

2. Centers for Disease Control and Prevention: http://www.cdc.gov/travel

3. International Society of Travel Medicine: http://www.istm.org

4. Shoreland, Inc.: http://www.travax.com (available by subscription only, which at the time of this writing, is $895 annually)

5. University of Washington Travel Medicine Clinic: http://hallhealth.washington.edu

6. U.S. Department of State: http://www.travel.state.gov

7. World Health Organization: http://www.who.org

Books

1. Arguin PM, Kozarsky PE, Navin AW, eds. *Health information for international travel.* 2005–06 edition. Philadelphia, PA: Elsevier Inc.; 2005–06.

2. Atkinson W, Hamborsky J, McIntyre L, et al., eds. *Epidemiology and prevention of vaccine-preventable diseases.* 8th ed. Washington, DC: Public Health Foundation; 2005.

3. Keystone JS, Kozarsky PE, Freedman DO, et al., eds. *Travel medicine.* Philadelphia, PA: Elsevier Limited; 2004.

4. Rose SR, Keystone JS. *International travel health guide 2006–2007*, 13th ed. Philadelphia, PA: Mosby, Inc.; 2006.

5. Thompson RF, ed. *Travel and routine immunizations.* 2005 ed. Milwaukee, WI: Shoreland, Inc.; 2005.

CASE STUDY

S: It is October 2006; the patient is a 67-year-old Ethiopian female referred to the pharmacist for a travel medicine consult. She comes in stating that she wants to get her "travel shots" today. She will be leaving for Ethiopia in 1 week and plans to travel for 6 months. She will stay mainly in Addis Ababa and may also go to Tigray via bus for a few days. She plans to visit her friends and family, will stay in their home, and does not plan any adventure travel. She came to the United States from Ethiopia last year and has not traveled internationally since then. She does not have records of immunization status and is unsure of her childhood diseases; however, she believes she had the polio vaccine before. She is on the state basic health plan.

PMH: Asthma, Type-2 diabetes, hyperlipidemia

Allergies: NKDA

Current medications:

Metformin 1000 mg bid

Glipizide 10 mg bid

Insulin NPH 15 units bid

Fluticasone/salmeterol 500/50 mcg 1 puff bid

Albuterol MDI prn

Atorvastatin 10 mg daily

Docusate 250 mg bid

Naproxen 250 mg bid prn pain

Immunization History: none documented; PPD negative last year

O:

Pertinent Labs:

  HbA1c: 9.8%

  BUN/Scr: 7/0.8

Lipids: TC 241, TG 192, HDL 45, LDL 126

AST/ALT: 19/37

Virology: Hep A and B antibody positive

A/P:

She is planning a trip to Ethiopia very soon for an extended duration. *She is, as with the majority of patients we see for travel consults, most interested in getting vaccinations; her "travel shots." She will be in the developing world for several months, has uncontrolled diabetes, hyperlipidemia, and asthma, and is on several chronic medications. Cardiovascular and respiratory diseases are probably her biggest health risks more so than risks from infection. She should be managed and educated accordingly. She should also be given her immunizations and anti-malarials as appropriate. A review of travel medicine resources on the date of service will help guide the recommendations, which are noted below.*

   1.   Routine immunizations. Provide vaccines for polio, varicella, tetanus-diphtheria, influenza, and pneumococcal. Counsel on indications and potential side effects of the vaccines. *She will be leaving very soon, so she may not be able to get adequate immunity before departure. However, she may receive some protection from at least the first dose of vaccinations and should be offered as appropriate. Since we are unsure of her vaccination history, all routine vaccinations should be considered. She thinks she had the polio vaccine, but without proof, it would be best to provide this vaccination for her because she is visiting an endemic area. She has immunity against hepatitis A and B, so there is no need to provide these vaccinations. Because she was born before 1957, she is presumed to have been exposed, so MMR vaccination is not recommended. She is unaware of her childhood disease history, but it is likely she was exposed to varicella, as she is from Ethiopia. Therefore, it is probably cost effective to order her varicella antibody status. However, we are short of time, so it would be best just to give her the immunization today as she has no contraindications. She is over 65 years old, so the tetanus-diphtheria-acellular pertussis is not indicated, but she should receive a dose of tetanus-diphtheria vaccine. She should also receive influenza vaccine (depending on availabil-*

ity) and pneumococcal vaccine. There is no contraindication to giving all vaccinations simultaneously today, although she is likely to be sore and may feel feverish.

2. Travel immunizations. In addition to the above immunizations, she should get typhoid and meningococcal vaccines. *Because of her time frame, she should get the injectable typhoid vaccine today because she won't have time to wait the full 8 days for the course of OTV.* She is a candidate for meningococcal vaccine and should receive this too. *Because of her age, Menactra™ is not indicated.* She should get yellow fever vaccine because she is going to an endemic area, although it is not a requirement. *It would be a requirement if she was planning to travel between Ethiopia and another yellow fever endemic area as part of her extended trip. Because this vaccine is not available at our institution, she is given information on where to get this vaccination locally. Although she denies planning camping or adventure travel, she is staying with family in the developing world, and if the family has pets or farms, rabies would potentially be a risk to her and the vaccine could be considered.*

3. Malaria chemoprophylaxis. There is no risk to her in Addis Ababa; however, she is tentatively planning travel to Tigray and she may be at risk for malaria there. Offer malaria chemoprophylaxis to take during the time she is in Tigray, and counsel on exactly when to start and stop taking it. Doxycycline, mefloquine, and atovaquone/ proguanil are options. Doxycycline would be recommended in her situation as it is the most cost-effective. Counsel on avoidance measures, including staying indoors at night and using impregnated clothing and netting as well as insect repellant containing DEET.

4. Diarrhea self-treatment. *Our institution does not routinely include this for pre-travel planning as discussed earlier. One could consider giving a prescription as listed in Table 19-2 and counseling accordingly.*

5. Education. Counsel on managing asthma and diabetes, especially with changing activity and diet. Educate about taking extra diabetes supplies; having treatment for hypoglycemia readily available, especially on the flight and during other travels; checking blood sugars more frequently; being mindful of proper hydration; and maintaining adequate foot care especially if walking a lot. Counsel on using sunscreen because glipizide can increase sun sensitivity as would doxycycline. Provide a prescription for compression stockings to wear on the plane and encourage her to have additional asthma rescue medication on hand. Counsel on additional topics pertinent to her destination, including food and water precautions, management of diarrhea, personal safety measures, avoidance of

freshwater swimming and contact with local animals, and when to seek medical help. *Although not often discussed with our low-income immigrants returning home in a short time frame, a discussion on travel insurance may be considered for other travelers, especially if they have multiple uncontrolled chronic conditions.*

6. Provide medication coordination to ensure adequate supply of necessary medications while traveling. *She will need medication for her diabetes and asthma while traveling. It would be best to continue her current regimen because its availability in Ethiopia is unknown. Since her insurance does not pay for more than a 30-day supply, she will have to pay up front for the remaining supply of medication to take with her. The atorvastatin would be very expensive, so we could consider changing to a generic statin at an equivalent dose (e.g., lovastatin 40 mg daily). Although given her short time frame, this is not very practical. Fluticasone/salmeterol would also be very expensive but it's the only viable option for her, especially with diabetes. If she is in agreement, consider holding her bowel and pain regimens because they are not as vital to her health.* Provide education on storing extra bottles of insulin that are not in use and on disposal of needles.

7. Follow-up. Encourage follow-up upon return. *At that time will need to assess for any illness during travel but, more importantly, she will need to resume her chronic medications and have her asthma and diabetes managed.* Place PPD and assess need for treatment with albendazole. Complete routine vaccination series, including tetanus-diphtheria. Consider completing polio vaccination series, especially if she plans future travel. Assess how well she utilized pre-travel planning and education given, and any barriers to implementation.

References

1. Ryan ET, Kain KC. Health advice and immunizations for travelers. *N Engl J Med.* 2000; 342:1716–25.

2. Freedman DO, Weld LH, Kozarsky PE, et al. Spectrum of disease and relation to place of exposure among ill returned travelers. *N Engl J Med.* 2006; 354:119–30.

3. Keystone JS, Kozarsky PE. Health advice for international travel. In: Guerrant RL, Walker DH, Weller PF, eds. *Essentials of tropical infectious diseases.* Philadelphia, PA: Churchill Livingstone; 2001:128–40.

4. Leder K, et al. Illness in travelers visiting friends and relatives: a review of the GeoSentinel Surveillance Network. *Clin Infect Dis.* 2006; 43:1185–93.

5. Angell SY, Cetron MS. Health disparities among travelers visiting friends and relatives abroad. *Ann Intern Med*. 2005; 142:67–72.

6. Bacaner N, Stauffer B, Boulware DR, et al. Travel medicine considerations for North American residents visiting friends and relatives. *JAMA*. 2004; 291:2856–64.

7. Jong EC. Immunizations for international travel. *Infect Dis Clin North Am*. 1998; 12:249–66.

8. Franco-Paredes C, Santos-Preciado JI. Problem pathogens: prevention of malaria in travelers. *Lancet Infect Dis*. 2006; 6:139–49.

9. Petersen E. Malaria chemoprophylaxis: when should we use it and what are the options? *Expert Rev Anti-infect Ther*. 2004; 2:119–32.

10. Steffen R. Epidemiology: morbidity and mortality in travelers. In: Keystone JS, Kozarsky PE, Freedman DO, et al., eds. *Travel medicine*. Philadelphia, PA: Elsevier Limited; 2004:5–12.

11. Chen LH, Wilson ME, Schlagenhauf P. Prevention of malaria in long-term travelers. *JAMA*. 2006; 296:2234–44.

12. Personal communication: Katie Lai, PharmD, CDE, BCPS. Clinical pharmacist in International Medicine Clinic 1997–2004. June 2006.

13. Hopewell CM, et al. Compression stockings for preventing deep vein thrombosis in airline passengers. *The Cochrane Library*. 2006; 2:1–30.

14. Meunnig P, Pallin D, Sell RL, et al. The cost effectiveness of strategies for the treatment of intestinal parasites in immigrants. *N Engl J Med*. 1999; 340:773–9.

Influenza and Pneumococcal Immunization

Heidi Sawyer

Influenza and pneumococcal illnesses cause a significant burden for Americans. For patients >65 years of age, pneumococcal disease—together with influenza—is the fifth most common cause of death.[1] Despite the effect of these diseases, vaccination among patients remains low with only 64% of non-institutionalized adults >65 years receiving influenza vaccine and 4% of adults >65 years receiving pneumococcal vaccine as of 1998.[2] These low rates have prompted immunizations to be a component of the national health objectives of Healthy People 2010, with the goal of increasing the vaccination rate to 90% for patients >65 years for both influenza and pneumococcal vaccines.[2] Pharmacists play a crucial role in making such vital vaccines widely available in the community. As of 2004, pharmacists are legally permitted to administer vaccines in 41 states.[2] This gives pharmacists a significant opportunity to prevent disease through immunization programs.

Influenza Vaccine

Indications[3]

1. Patients at increased risk for complications of influenza. Vaccination with inactivated vaccine is recommended.

    a. Age >65 years

    b. Patients with chronic disorders of the pulmonary or cardiovascular systems (includes asthma but not hypertension)

    c. Patients with required regular medical follow-up or hospitalization during the preceding year due to chronic metabolic diseases (diabetes mellitus, renal dysfunction, hemoglobinopathies, and immunosuppression)

d. Patients with any condition that can compromise respiratory function or the handling of respiratory secretions or that can increase the risk for aspiration (cognitive dysfunction, spinal cord injuries, seizure disorders, or other neuromuscular disorders)

e. Children 6 months–18 years who are receiving long-term aspirin therapy and are at increased risk of Reye's syndrome

f. Children 6–23 months old

g. Women who are pregnant during the influenza season

h. Residents of nursing homes or chronic care facilities

2. Patients at increased risk for clinic, emergency room, or hospital visits due to influenza. Vaccination with inactivated vaccine is recommended.[3]

a. Patients 50–64 years old (increased prevalence of high-risk conditions in this age group)

b. Children age 24–59 months old

3. Persons who can transmit influenza to those at high risk. Inactivated vaccine is recommended for those in contact with severely immunocompromised patients. All others may receive live attenuated influenza vaccine (LAIV) if appropriate.[3]

a. Health care workers

b. Employees of assisted living and other residences for patients in high-risk groups

c. Caregivers and household contacts of patients in high-risk groups

d. Household contacts and out-of-home caregivers for children 0–59 months old

4. General population. Depending on vaccine availability and exclusion criteria, influenza vaccine is available to any patient who requests it.

Exclusion Criteria

1. General screening for exclusion criteria for all immunizations:

a. Complete questionnaire provided by Immunization Action Coalition (www.immunize.org/catg.d/p4065scr.pdf). The questionnaire discusses the role of minor illness, allergies, reactions to vaccines, immunosuppression, blood transfusions, pregnancy, and vaccine interactions.

2. Exclusion criteria for inactivated influenza vaccine:[4]

a. Anaphylactic hypersensitivity to eggs or other components of the vaccine

b. Patients <6 months old

3. Exclusion criteria for LAIV:[4]

    a. Persons <5 years or $\geq$50 years

    b. Patients with asthma, reactive airways disease, or other chronic pulmonary or cardiovascular disorders; patients with chronic medical conditions such as metabolic diseases (diabetes, renal dysfunction, hemoglobinopathies); and patients with known or suspected immunodeficiency diseases

    c. Children up to 18 years of age who are receiving aspirin or other salicylates

    d. Patients with a history of Guillain-Barré Syndrome

    e. Pregnant women

    f. Patients with a history of hypersensitivity, including anaphylaxis to any components of LAIV or to eggs

    g. Those in close contact with severely immunocompromised patients (e.g., stem-cell transplant patients during the time that the patient is in a protected environment)

Management of Immunization

1. General risks of immunization: local reactions, fainting, and anaphylaxis

    a. Local reactions include soreness, redness, and itching at the site of injection. This can be managed with a cold compress, an analgesic, or antipruritic medication. Other local reactions include minor bleeding at the site of the injection, which can be managed with a bandage.

    b. For further information on the treatment of local reactions, fainting, and anaphylaxis, refer to www.immunize.org/catg.d/p3082.pdf.

2. Influenza vaccine

    a. Treatment options for prevention and treatment of influenza

        i. Prevention via vaccine (inactivated or LAIV)

        ii. Prevention with antivirals during the influenza season or during specific epidemics or treatment with antivirals at the time of diagnosis

          • *Note*: amantadine and rimantidine are no longer recommended for prevention or treatment of influenza A due to increased levels of resistance.[3]

          • Oseltamivir or zanamivir remain viable options for prevention or treatment of influenza A.[3]

    b. Benefits of influenza vaccine: prevention of influenza disease and complications

        i. Effectiveness depends on age and immunocompetence of the patient, as well as the match between the actual virus in circulation and the influenza vaccine[4] (**Table 20-1**)

Table 20-1. Efficacy of Influenza Vaccine[5]

Types of Vaccines	Efficacy of Vaccine	Comments
Inactivated Influenza Vaccine		
<65 years	70–90% protective against influenza	May decrease to 52% for healthy adults and 38% for patients with one high-risk condition if vaccine poorly matched[5]
Children	77–91%	May decrease to 49% if vaccine poorly matched
≥65 years	58% for non-nursing home patients 30–40% for nursing home patients	30–70% effective vs. influenza-related hospitalization for pneumonia or influenza for non-nursing home patients 50–60% effective vs. influenza-related hospitalization for nursing home patients
LAIV		
Healthy Children	87–93%	May decrease to 86–87% effective if poorly matched
Healthy Adults	85%	Effectiveness may decrease if poorly matched. One study found 26% decrease in febrile URI[5]

c. Risks of inactivated influenza vaccine:[4]

　i. Soreness at the vaccination site <2 days in 10–64% of patients

　ii. Fever, malaise, and myalgia may occur post-vaccination, most often in patients receiving vaccine for the first time

　iii. Allergic reactions (hives, angioedema, allergic asthma, and systemic anaphylaxis) due to egg allergies

　　• Screen all patients to prevent administration to those with egg allergy. Be prepared to treat anaphylactic reactions with epinephrine 1:1000 (via Epipen® or ampule), monitor vital signs, and administer CPR if needed. (See www.immunize.org/catg.d/p3082.pdf for further information.)

　　• Complete Vaccine Adverse Effect Reporting System (VAERS) form for any adverse event. Form is available at www.vaers.org.

　iv. Thimerosal. Some inactivated influenza vaccine products contain 25 mcg of mercury (as the preservative thimerosal) per 0.5 mL of vaccine. Inactivated vaccine is also available as a thimerosal-free product. This product is recommended for infants and pregnant women.

　v. Guillain-Barré Syndrome (GBS). GBS was linked to vaccination during the swine flu epidemic of 1976. Since that time, the incidence of patients receiving influenza vaccine has been one additional case greater than the background incidence of 10–20 cases/1 million adults. Highest risk is within 6 weeks of vaccination.

d.   Risks of LAIV in healthy adults[4] (**Table 20-2**)

Table 20-2. Side Effects of LAIV[5]

	Side Effects with LAIV	Side Effects with Placebo
Cough	13.9%	10.8%
Runny nose	44.5%	27.1%
Sore throat	27.8%	17.1%
Chills	8.6%	6.0%
Tiredness/weakness	25.7%	12.6%

e.   Influenza vaccine patient education:

   i.   Lack of risk of inactivated influenza vaccine causing influenza

   ii. Risk of upper respiratory infection occurring post-vaccination if a respiratory virus is already present at the time of vaccination

   iii. Importance of preventing influenza and related complications, especially in high-risk populations

Goals of Therapy

1.   Provide target doses of inactivated influenza vaccine[4] to appropriate patients (**Table 20-3**).

Table 20-3. Target Doses of Inactivated Influenza Vaccine[5]

Age Group	Dose	Number of Doses	Route
6–35 months	0.25 mL	2 doses 1 month apart if first use, otherwise 1 dose	IM
3–8 years	0.5 mL	2 doses 1 month apart if first use, otherwise 1 dose	IM
>9 years	0.5 mL	1	IM

2.   Provide target doses of LAIV[1] to appropriate patients (**Table 20-4**).

Table 20-4. Target Doses of LAIV[5]

Age Group	Dose	Number of Doses	Route
5–8 years	0.25 mL sprayed into each nostril	2 doses 6–10 weeks apart if first use, otherwise 1 dose	Nasal
9–49 years	0.25 mL sprayed into each nostril	1	Nasal

Pneumococcal Vaccine

Indications[5]

1. Age >65 years
2. Patients with chronic illnesses:
   a. Chronic cardiac disease
   b. Chronic pulmonary disease (excluding asthma)
   c. Diabetes mellitus
   d. Chronic liver disease, including those caused by alcohol abuse, such as cirrhosis
   e. Chronic renal disease or nephrotic syndrome
   f. Functional or anatomic asplenia (e.g., sickle cell disease or splenectomy)
   g. Immunosuppressive conditions (e.g., congenital immunodeficiency, HIV, leukemia, lymphoma, Hodgkin's disease, multiple myeloma, generalized malignancy, and organ or bone marrow transplant)
   h. Chemotherapy with alkylating agents, antimetabolites, or high-dose long-term corticosteroids
   i. Patients with cochlear implants
   j. Patients living in special environments or social settings, including Alaska natives and certain American Indian tribes, residents of nursing homes, or other long-term care facilities
3. Indications for revaccination with pneumococcal vaccine[5]
   a. For patients >65 years, a one-time revaccination is recommended if age <65 years at the time of the primary pneumococcal vaccine and 5 years has elapsed since the primary vaccination.
   b. One-time revaccination after 5 years is recommended for those with the following medical conditions:
      i. Chronic renal failure or nephrotic syndrome
      ii. Functional or anatomic asplenia
      iii. Immunosuppressive conditions (see list above)
      iv. Chemotherapy with alkylating agents, antimetabolites, or high-dose long-term corticosteroids

Exclusion Criteria

1. General screening for exclusion criteria for all immunizations:
   a. Complete questionnaire provided by Immunization Action Coalition (www.immunize.org/catg.d/p4065scr.pdf). The questionnaire discusses the role of minor illness, allergies, reactions to vaccines, immunosuppression, blood transfusions, pregnancy, and vaccine interactions.

2. Exclusion criteria for pneumococcal vaccine:

    a. Allergic reaction to the vaccine or its components. *Note*: pneumococcal vaccine does not contain eggs.

Management of Immunization

1. General risks of immunization: local reactions, fainting, and anaphylaxis

    a. Local reactions include soreness, redness, and itching at the site of injection. This can be managed with a cold compress, an analgesic, and anti-pruritic medication. Other local reactions include minor bleeding at the site of the injection, which can be managed with a bandage.

    b. For further information on the treatment of local reactions, fainting, and anaphylaxis, refer to www.immunize.org/catg.d/p3082.pdf.

2. Treatment options for pneumococcal disease

    a. Prevention via vaccine

    b. Treatment of pneumococcal disease as appropriate at the time of diagnosis

3. Benefits: 23 valent pneumococcal polysaccharide vaccine (PPV23) used in adults protects against 88% of pneumococcal disease. Cross reaction also occurs with several other subtypes and provides 8% additional coverage.[6]

4. Risks: side effects of pneumococcal vaccine (**Table 20-5**)

Table 20-5. Side Effects of Pneumococcal Vaccine[6]

Reaction	Frequency
Injection site reactions	30–50% (greater after the first injection)
Fever, myalgia	<1%

5. Pneumococcal vaccine patient education

    a. Lack of risk of inactivated pneumococcal vaccine causing pneumococcal disease

    b. Importance of preventing pneumococcal disease and related complications, especially in high-risk populations

Goal of Therapy

1. Provide target doses (0.5 mL intramuscularly or subcutaneously) of pneumococcal vaccine (PPV23) to appropriate patients.[7]

Other Vaccines

Pharmacists may be involved in providing immunizations beyond the influenza and pneumococcal vaccines listed above. For further information about the indications of other vaccines, see the following references:

1. Adult immunization schedule: http://www.cdc.gov/nip/recs/adult-schedule.pdf
2. Childhood immunization schedule: http://www.cdc.gov/nip/recs/child-schedule-color-print.pdf

Clinical Pharmacy Goals

1. Offer vaccination to all appropriate patients
   a. Advertise services to patients, including hours and costs (e.g., reminder postcards)
   b. Screen patients to identify those not eligible for vaccination (sample screening questionnaire: www.immunize.org/catg.d/p4065scr.pdf)
   c. Identify patients most in need of vaccination by screening for those at high risk for influenza or pneumococcal disease
2. Educate patients
   a. Discuss vaccine side effects (see above)
   b. Reassure fears of contracting influenza or pneumococcal disease from inactivated vaccine
   c. Provide CDC vaccine information sheets (see www.cdc.gov/nip/publications/vis/)
   d. Offer consent forms for vaccination
      i. Generic forms: http://www.immunizeseniors.org/website/p1I.htm
      ii. Influenza in Washington state: http://www.doh.wa.gov/cfh/Immunize/documents/348-054_flu.pdf
      iii. Pneumococcal in Washington state: http://www.doh.wa.gov/cfh/Immunize/documents/348-056_pneupoly.pdf
   e. Provide a record of vaccine administration for patient (sample: http://www3.doh.wa.gov/here/materials/PDFs/15_ImmuCard_E06L.pdf)
3. Store and handle vaccines appropriately in the pharmacy
   a. Refrigerate (including influenza and pneumococcal) or freeze (including FluMist©) as appropriate (sample refrigerator monitoring form: http://www.doh.wa.gov/cfh/immunize/documents/tempmontlog03.pdf)
   b. Rotate stock, including checking expiration dates, and order sensibly
   c. Record administration of vaccine in pharmacy
      i. Sample: www.doh.wa.gov/cfh/immunize/documents/vacadminrecord.pdf
   d. Bill vaccines to third-party insurance, as appropriate
   e. Establish prescriptive authority agreement with provider (sample: http://apps.leg.wa.gov/WAC/default.aspx?cite=246-863-100)

4. Administration of vaccines

   a. Attain vaccine certification in your state; American Pharmacists Association (APhA) began a national immunization training program in 1996

   b. Be familiar with the legal requirements of vaccine administration in your state

   c. Utilize proper technique for intramuscular injections (diagram: http://www.health.state.mn.us/divs/idepc/newsletters/gys/admim.pdf)

Outcome Measures

1. Process measures: Improve percentage of eligible patients receiving influenza vaccine and pneumococcal vaccine; provide cost-effective immunization services and third-party insurance billing, as appropriate.

2. Health outcome measures: Improve prevention of pneumococcal and influenza disease and associated complications such as pneumonia, hospitalization, and death.

Resources

Patient Information Resources

1. CDC, influenza vaccine information: http://www.cdc.gov/flu/

2. CDC, national immunization program: http://www.cdc.gov/nip/

3. WebMD, adult immunizations: http://www.webmd.com/content/article/123/115060.htm

Provider Information Resources

1. Immunization Action Coalition: http://www.immunize.org

2. Vaccine Adverse Event Reporting System: http://www.vaers.org

3. NIP/CDC adult vaccination schedule: http://www.cdc.gov/nip/recs/adult-schedule.pdf

4. CDC guidelines for vaccinating pregnant women: http://www.cdc.gov/nip/publications/preg_guide.pdf

References

1. Grabenstein JD, Raney EC. ASHP guidelines on the pharmacist's role in immunization: developed through the ASHP Council on Professional Affairs and approved by the ASHP Board of Directors on May 31, 2003. *Am J Health-Syst Pharm*. 2003; 60:1371–7.

2. Sokos DR. Pharmacists' role in increasing pneumococcal and influenza vaccination. *Am J Health-Syst Pharm*. 2005; 62:367–77.

3. CDC. Prevention and control of influenza: recommendations of the Advisory Committee on Immunization Practices (ACIP). *MMWR*. 2006; 55 (No. RR 10).

4. CDC. Prevention and control of influenza: recommendations of the Advisory Committee on Immunization Practices (ACIP). *MMWR*. 2005; 54 (No. RR-8).

5. CDC. Recommended adult immunization schedule—United States. October 2006– September 2007. *MMWR*. 2006; 55:Q1–4.

6. Atkinson W, Hamborsky J, McIntyre L, et al, eds. *Epidemiology and prevention of vaccine-preventable diseases*, 8th ed. Washington, DC: Public Health Foundation; 2005.

7. Thompson RF, ed. *Travel and routine immunizations: a practical guide for the medical office*. Milwaukee, WI: Shoreland, Inc.; 2005.

Refill Authorization

Manzi Berlin, Carol Johnson

The Refill Authorization Center (RAC) was established to provide uninterrupted chronic medication therapy to patients seen in all primary care clinics and select specialty care clinics. The RAC is staffed by clinical pharmacists and one pharmacy technician, who provides clerical support services. The pharmacists' refill authorization decisions are based on disease management protocols developed in concert with state pharmacist prescriptive authority guidelines. The protocols are approved by the clinic medical directors and the state board of pharmacy on a biennial basis.

Indications

Patients utilizing the RAC must be in the care of a participating provider and be seen routinely for ongoing medical care. Requests received for patients not eligible for the service or not meeting RAC criteria are forwarded to the appropriate clinic or provider. In addition, the requesting pharmacy is given the correct contact information for future reference.

Management

Patients are able to access the RAC in a variety of ways. The preferred method is for the patient to contact the pharmacy and request a faxed, formal request for medication refills. Many pharmacies have interactive voice response (IVR) technologies that automatically generate a refill request form when a prescription has no remaining refills. The fax process helps to assure that all information regarding the prescription is available to the reviewing pharmacist: identity of the patient, date of birth, medication, current dose, prescriber, and refill history. Alternatively, patients may contact the RAC directly by telephone and leave a voice message. This often requires a follow-up telephone call to the patient to retrieve missing, but pertinent, information. Patients who contact their prescriber regarding refills are transferred to the RAC voice messaging service. Many clinics provide their patients with educational tools such as flyers and refrigerator magnets to assist them in accessing the refill center.

Goals of Service

The RAC pharmacist reviews the patient medication profile for accuracy, potential drug interactions, and duplication of therapy. By utilizing approved protocols, such as the example shown in **Figure 21-1**, providers are confident that the refill authorization process is standardized and consistent.[2] Pharmacists document all refill authorization activity in the electronic medical record. When necessary, communication with providers is accomplished through a secure e-mail system or by direct telephone contact. The primary service goal is to enhance clinic efficiency by freeing both providers and clinic support staff from managing prescription refills.

Clinical Goals

The RAC endeavors to maximize medication safety, efficacy, and adherence. This objective is met when chronic medication therapy is provided to all patients in a timely manner and there is no disruption in therapy. The goal is further advanced by the pharmacists' critical review of all pertinent aspects of medication therapy.[3] The pharmacist provides the key link among the patient, prescriber, and dispensing pharmacist. Goals are met through

1. Uninterrupted access to chronic medications within 24–48 hours of receipt of request.

2. Continuity of care for patients seen in multiple clinics within a health system.

3. Appropriate monitoring of medications and disease states by recommending appropriate laboratory testing and follow-up appointments, identifying issues with adherence or duplicate therapy, and clarifying medication dosage questions.

4. Therapeutic substitution under provider-approved protocols to meet the formulary requirements of third-party insurers and the health system.

Outcome Measures

Monthly statistics are reported reflecting the number of patients served and the number of prescriptions processed. Monthly quality assurance reports are generated to identify challenges and subsequent solutions. When problems are identified, every attempt is made to take corrective action and to maintain effective communication with providers.[4]

References

1. UW Medicine Refill Authorization Center. Medication Refill Protocol (125 pages). Seattle, WA: University of Washington Medicine Department of Pharmacy Services. October 15, 2006.

2. Riege VJ. A Patient Safety Program and Research Evaluation of U.S. Navy Pharmacy Refill Clinic. Available at http://www.ahrq.gov/downloads/pub/advances/vol1/Reige.pdf. Accessed May 10, 2006.

3. Bobrt KF, Purohit AA. Refilling prescription and physician consent. *Contemp Pharm Pract.* 1982; 5(2):80–4.

4. D'Achille KM, Swanson LN, Hill ET Jr. Pharmacist-managed patient assessment and medication refill clinic. *Am J Hosp Pharm.* 1978; 35(1):66–70.

Methotrexate

UW MEDICINE DEPARTMENT OF PHARMACY
Medication Refill Protocol
October 15, 2006

Endocrinology / Rheumatology:

A. Determine from the chart or electronic medical record:

1. Indication of medication
2. Strength and dosage of medication
3. Date of last physician/provider appointment
4. Date of next appointment from physician/provider instructions
5. Quantity of medication to last until next appointment or 12 months from last annual appointment if "PRN"
6. Other medications taken concurrently; check for drug interactions
7. Last hepatic, hematologic, and renal monitoring (see below); record on Refill Request Form

B. If information in "A" is available in the chart or MINDSCAPE:

1. Authorize the refill
2. Update the Medication List in electronic medical record, then record refill

C. If information in "A" is not available in the electronic medical record, telephone the patient for the information, and, in addition, check for:

Figure 21-1 (continued on next page)

Renal Monitoring:

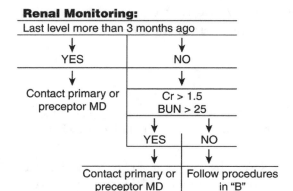

Hepatic Monitoring:

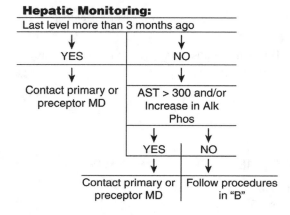

Hematologic Monitoring:

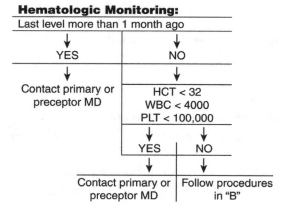

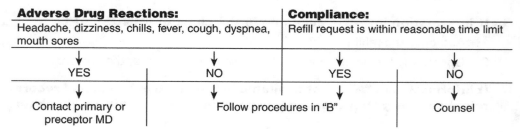

Figure 21-1. (continued)

Quality Improvement Mechanisms

Privileging Process for Pharmacists

Cynthia A. Clegg

The Privileging Process

As pharmacists assume more responsibility for direct patient care, organizations and payers will require pharmacists to participate in institutional privileging. The privileging process is used in health care organizations to authorize practitioners to provide specific patient care services within their institution. It is the mechanism used to assure that the individual is qualified and competent to provide those patient care services being authorized.

Terminology within the credentialing or privileging process can be confusing. Therefore, we will use terminology consistent with the definitions developed by the Council on Credentialing in Pharmacy.[1] A glossary of these terms can be found in **Appendix 22-1**.

The Joint Commission® has specific requirements with regard to privileging policy and procedure that must be delineated in the organization's medical staff bylaws. Institutions may have slightly different privileging processes, but all are based on the patient care standards of the granting organization and scope of practice laws and regulations. In 2004 *AJHP* published an excellent primer on credentialing and privileging for pharmacists, which describes processes, identifies resources, and provides case studies on this topic.[2]

Most organizations have a standing committee charged with the granting of privileges. The Department of Pharmacy should engage with the Credentialing Committee to establish the scope of practice and privileging requirements for specific clinical pharmacy practitioners. The process begins with an application for clinical privileges. Generally, this includes a comprehensive list of the information needed by the committee to approve privileges. The pharmacist must show evidence of graduation from an accredited college of pharmacy, current state licensure, and added credentials deemed necessary for patient care activities, which may include accredited residency training and board certification. The committee members review the application in light of the scope of practice documents and the organizational privileges being requested. Privileges are granted for a defined period of time, and renewal requires ongoing competency assessments that are submitted to the Credentialing Committee on a regularly scheduled basis.

Organizational application packets are relatively standard across the professions, although credentials specific to pharmacy practice should be included. A scope of practice document is unique to each specialty practice. A sample scope of practice document for clinical pharmacy specialists practicing in a primary care setting under liberal collaborative drug therapy management (CDTM) agreements is included below.

Scope of Practice: Ambulatory Clinical Pharmacy Specialists

Purpose

Identify scope-of-practice privileges for the clinical pharmacy specialists (CPS) at Harborview Medical Center (HMC), and define criteria for the qualifications for these privileges. The CPS will be qualified and authorized to perform specific clinical duties to ensure that cost-effective, high-quality health care and appropriate pharmaceutical care are provided to patients.

Policy

Scope-of-practice guidelines for CPS shall be delineated in writing and will follow established protocols approved by the HMC Clinic Medical Directors, Associate Medical Director for Ambulatory Care Services, Medical Director, and the Washington State Board of Pharmacy.

Qualifications

The CPS is trained in clinical therapeutics, pharmacokinetics, and pharmacology. He or she is a master's or Doctor of Pharmacy (Pharm.D.) graduate and has completed an accredited pharmacy residency and specialty residency in primary care; the CPS is a specialty board-certified pharmacist or has equivalent education, training, and experience functioning as a clinical pharmacist. The HMC Credentialing Committee privileges all ambulatory CPSs practicing at Harborview Medical Center.

Structure and Process

In most cases, the CPS works in the clinic's provider room to facilitate consultations between the CPS and attending physicians, medical residents, mid-level practitioners, and other providers. The CPS shall provide consultations and accept referrals from medical staff. The role of the CPS differs with attending physicians and medical residents. In the case of medical residents who are in training to manage various patient care issues, the CPS shall offer consultation (education) on medication therapy management.

In the case of attending physicians, the CPS shall provide consultation services and accept referrals for therapeutic disease state management activities that require intensive medication dosage titration, management, and follow-up. In the vast majority of cases, patients referred to the CPS are identified as "high risk" for drug-related problems. These risks include:

- Five or more medications in a regimen
- Twelve or more doses per day
- A medication regimen that changes often
- Three or more concurrent disease states
- A history of non-compliance
- The presence of drugs that require therapeutic drug monitoring[3]

Key Functions

The CPS collaborates with physicians to provide safe, evidence-based, cost-effective medication therapy management that improves a patient's health-related quality of life through the following actions:

- Conducts comprehensive appraisals of patients' health status by taking health and drug histories and performing physical examinations necessary to assess drug therapy.
- Documents relevant findings of a patient's health status in his or her medical record.
- Evaluates drug therapy through direct patient care involvement with clinical assessment as well as subjective and objective findings related to patients' responses to drug therapy and communicates and documents the findings and recommendations to appropriate individuals and in the medical record.
- Develops, documents, and executes therapeutic plans utilizing the most effective, least toxic, and most economic medication treatments as per national, pharmacy and therapeutics committee, or HMC-specific guidelines or protocols including the preferred drug formulary.
- Orders and analyzes laboratory and diagnostic test data so as to modify drug therapy and dosing, as necessary.

- Implements medications, including initiation, continuation, discontinuation, and therapy alterations, based upon established formulary or protocols.

- Provides ongoing primary care for chronic stable or minor acute health problems, as delineated in protocols and procedures, and assists in the management of medical emergencies, adverse drug reactions, and acute and chronic disease states.

- Provides patient and health care professional education and medication education.

- Evaluates and documents patients' and caregivers' ability to understand medication instructions and provides oral and written counseling on their medications.

- Documents relevant findings in the patients' medical records.

- Conducts and coordinates research drug investigations and research under FDA guidelines and regulations and approval by appropriate local officials.

- Completes facility billing for all CPS visits.

- Administers medication according to pre-established protocols.

- Identifies and takes specific corrective action for drug-induced problems.

- Serves as a clinical manager of drug-related programs in clinics in conjunction with the attending physician.

Supervision

The ultimate responsibility for CPS staff rests with the Assistant Director of Ambulatory Pharmacy Services; however, a collegial relationship with mutual consultation and referral exists between physicians and the CPS. Consultation with the physician or referring practitioner is outlined, and co-signature is required for practice outside approved procedures and protocols. The CPS will provide patient care as a non-physician clinician. A physician is available at all times by telephone or in person for consultation. Periodic chart and peer reviews by pharmacy and medical colleagues and annual evaluations provide ongoing quality assurance and medication-use evaluation. The CPS practices are included in the medication-use evaluation process.

Patient Outcomes

When possible, HMC-specific patient outcomes will be assessed using the Value Compass (Harborview's version of the balanced scorecard) methodology. When this is not possible, evidence-based literature on the effectiveness of clinical pharmacy services shall be used to predict the economic, clinical, operational, and humanistic outcomes of the service.

An excellent resource for information regarding privileging and credentialing can by found on the ASHP website at: http://www.ashp.org/s_ashp/quart2c.asp?CID=1229&DID=1271.

Summary

It is particularly important for pharmacists practicing under CDTM agreements to undergo privileging within their organization. It serves to define their role in direct patient care as part of the health care team, establishes their competency in and accountability for providing these services, provides a framework for ongoing competency assessment, and supports billing for services provided.

References

1. Council on Credentialing in Pharmacy. Credentialing in pharmacy. *Am J Health-Syst Pharm.* 2001; 58:69–76.

2. Galt KA. Credentialing and privileging for pharmacists. *Am J Health-Syst Pharm.* 2004; 61:661–70.

3. Koecheler JA, Abramowitz PW, Swim SE, et al. Indicators for the selection of ambulatory patients who warrant pharmacist monitoring. *Am J Hosp Pharm.* 1989; 46:729–32.

Appendix 22-1: Credentialing in Pharmacy

■

SPECIAL FEATURE

Credentialing in pharmacy

THE COUNCIL ON CREDENTIALING IN PHARMACY

Am J Health-Syst Pharm. 2001; 58:69-76

INTRODUCTION

Pharmacist credentialing has become a topic of important discussions in the profession of pharmacy in recent years. These discussions, inherently complex, have sometimes been further complicated by the lack of a common lexicon. The situation is understandable. Many different words are used to describe the process by which pharmacists are educated, trained, licensed, and otherwise recognized for their competence and achievements. Many different organizations—public and private—are involved in assessing pharmacists' knowledge and skills, granting credentials, and accrediting programs and institutions.

Purpose of This Paper

The purpose of this paper is to create a common frame of reference and understanding for discussions concerning pharmacist credentialing. It begins with definitions of several terms that are essential to any discussion of credentialing. This is followed by a short section highlighting the importance of credentialing to pharmacists. The next three sections, which form the body of the paper, discuss in detail the three types of credentials that pharmacists may earn:

- Credentials needed to prepare for practice (i.e., academic degrees),
- Credentials needed to enter practice (i.e., licensure) and to update professional knowledge and skills (i.e., relicensure) under state law, and

- Credentials that pharmacists voluntarily earn to document their specialized or advanced knowledge and skills (i.e., postgraduate degrees, certificates, certification).

Each of these sections contains, as applicable, information about the credential awarded, the training site, whether the credential is voluntary or mandatory, the credentialing body, and the agency that accredits the program. Particular attention is given to pharmacist certification programs, an area that has engendered much of the current interest in pharmacist credentialing.

The paper also includes a brief section on credentialing of pharmacy supportive personnel. It concludes with two appendices. Appendix A contains a comprehensive glossary of key terms relating to pharmacist credentialing. Appendix B is an alphabetical list of organizations involved in pharmacist credentialing and program accreditation. The list contains names, addresses, and uniform resource locators (URLs).

Council on Credentialing in Pharmacy

"Credentialing in Pharmacy" has

been created by the Council on Credentialing in Pharmacy (CCP), a coalition of 11 national pharmacy organizations founded in 1999 to provide leadership, standards, public information, and coordination for professional voluntary credentialing programs in pharmacy. Founding members of the CCP include the following organizations:

- Academy of Managed Care Pharmacy
- American Association of Colleges of Pharmacy
- American College of Apothecaries
- American College of Clinical Pharmacy
- American Council on Pharmaceutical Education
- American Pharmaceutical Association
- American Society of Consultant Pharmacists
- American Society of Health-System Pharmacists
- Board of Pharmaceutical Specialties
- Commission for Certification in Geriatric Pharmacy
- Pharmacy Technician Certification Board

SIX ESSENTIAL DEFINITIONS

Discussions of credentialing are often complicated by a lack of common understanding of key terms and the contexts in which they are used. To clarify these misunderstandings, one must first distinguish between processes (e.g., credentialing) and titles (a credential). Distinctions must also be made between processes that focus on individuals (e.g., credentialing and certification) and those that

A white paper prepared by the Council on Credentialing in Pharmacy (www.pharmacycredentialing.org), 2215 Constitution Avenue, NW, Washington, DC 20037, September 2000.

focus on organizations (accreditation). Finally, it is essential to understand that for practicing pharmacists, some credentials are required (e.g., an academic degree or a state license) while others are earned voluntarily (e.g., certification).

Beyond these distinctions, it is also necessary to understand the definitions of the words that commonly come up in discussions of credentialing and to be able to distinguish the sometimes-subtle differences among them. A comprehensive glossary of such words and their definitions appears in Appendix A. The following definitions are provided here because an understanding of these terms is a prerequisite to any meaningful discussion of credentialing in pharmacy.

- A *credential* is documented evidence of a pharmacist's qualifications. Pharmacist credentials include diplomas, licenses, certificates, and certifications. These credentials are reflected in a variety of abbreviations that pharmacists place after their names (e.g., Pharm.D. for "doctor of pharmacy," an earned academic degree; R.Ph. for "registered pharmacist," which indicates state licensure; and acronyms such as BCNSP for "Board-Certified Nutrition Support Pharmacist," which indicates that an individual has demonstrated advanced knowledge or skill in a specialized area of pharmacy).
- *Credentialing* is the process by which an organization or institution obtains, verifies, and assesses a pharmacist's qualifications to provide patient care services.
- *Accreditation* is the process by which a private association, organization, or government agency, after initial and periodic evaluations, grants recognition to an organization that has met certain established criteria.
- A *certificate* is a document issued to a pharmacist upon successful completion of the predetermined level of performance of a certificate training program or of a pharmacy residency or fellowship.

- A *statement of continuing-education credit* is a document issued to a pharmacist upon participation in an accredited continuing-education program.
- *Certification* is a voluntary process by which a nongovernmental agency or an association grants recognition to a pharmacist who has met certain predetermined qualifications specified by that organization. This formal recognition is granted to designate to the public that this pharmacist has attained the requisite level of knowledge, skill, or experience in a well-defined, often specialized, area of the total discipline. Certification usually requires initial assessment and periodic reassessments of the individual's qualifications.

IMPORTANCE OF CREDENTIALS IN PHARMACY

"Credential" and "credentialing," like the words "creed" and "credence," derive from the Latin verb *credere*, which means "to trust," "to entrust," or "to believe." A pharmacist's credentials are indicators that he or she holds the qualifications needed to practice the profession of pharmacy and is therefore worthy of the trust of patients, of other health care professionals, and of society as a whole.

In the profession of pharmacy, the interest in credentials has been catalyzed in recent years by several factors. First among them is the pace of change and the increasing complexity of health care. A second factor is the pharmacist's expanding clinical role. Interest in credentialing has likewise been stimulated by the growing trend toward specialization in pharmacy practice and by the need to document the pharmacist's ability to provide specialty care.

Another contributing factor has been the need to help ensure lifelong competence in a rapidly changing, technologically complex field. The need to provide a means of standardization of practice has also had a role. Such a motivation was key, for example, to the development of the Feder-

al Credentialing Program, which is creating a national database of health professionals that will include pharmacists.

Finally, economic realities enter the picture. Pharmacists who are providing cognitive services or specialized care need to be reimbursed for the services they provide. Payers rightfully demand validation that pharmacists are qualified to provide such services. Credentials, and in many cases, more specifically, certification, can help provide the documentation that Medicare and Medicaid, managed care organizations, and other third-party payers require of pharmacists today and in the future.

OVERVIEW OF CREDENTIALING IN PHARMACY

Introduction

Pharmacist credentials may be divided into three fundamental types.

- The first type—college and university degrees—is awarded to mark the successful completion of a pharmacist's academic training and education.
- The second type—licensure and relicensure—is an indication that the pharmacist has met minimum requirements set by the state in which he or she intends to practice.
- The third type of credential—which may include advanced degrees and certificates—is awarded to pharmacy practitioners who have completed programs of various types that are intended to develop and enhance their knowledge and skills, or who have successfully documented an advanced level of knowledge and skill through an assessment process.

These three paths to pharmacist credentialing are illustrated in Figure 1. The sections that follow provide information on each of the credentials offered in pharmacy, the credentialing or accreditation body involved, whether the credential is mandatory or voluntary, and other related information.

Figure 1. U.S. pharmacy credentials and oversight bodies. ACPE = American Council on Pharmaceutical Education, ASHP = American Society of Health-System Pharmacists, NABP = National Association of Boards of Pharmacy, ACCP = American College of Clinical Pharmacy, AACP = American Association of Colleges of Pharmacy, BPS = Board of Pharmaceutical Specialties, CCGP = Commission for Certification in Geriatric Pharmacy, NISPC = National Institute for Standards in Pharmacist Credentialing, PTCB = Pharmacy Technician Certification Board.

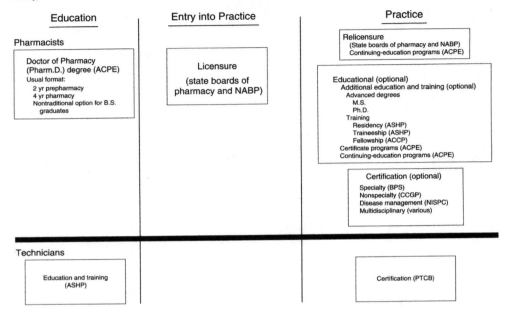

Preparing for the Pharmacy Profession

- Credential earned: Bachelor of Science degree in Pharmacy; Doctor of Pharmacy degree
- Credential awarded by: School or college of pharmacy
- Accreditation body for professional programs in pharmacy: American Council on Pharmaceutical Education (ACPE). The U.S. Department of Education has recognized the ACPE accreditation of the professional degree program in pharmacy.

Until July 1, 2000, an individual who wished to become a pharmacist could enroll in a program of study that would lead to one of two degrees: a bachelor of science degree in pharmacy (B.S. Pharm. or Pharm. B.S.) or a doctor of pharmacy (Pharm.D.) degree.

As of 1998, two-thirds of all stu-dents studying in professional programs in pharmacy were enrolled in Pharm.D. programs. The Pharm.D. degree became the sole degree accredited by ACPE for pharmacists' entry into practice in the United States, as of July 1, 2000, with the institution of new ACPE professional program accreditation standards. Pharm.D. programs typically take six years to complete and generally involve two years of preprofessional coursework and four years of professional education. A few programs offer the professional education over three years of full-time education.

B.S.-level pharmacists who have been in the workforce may also return to a college or school of pharmacy to earn the Pharm.D. degree. These programs, which are tailored to the individual's background and experience, may follow "nontraditional" pathways; however, they must produce the same educational outcomes as does the entry-level Pharm.D. degree.

State boards of pharmacy require a Pharm.D. or B.S. degree from a program approved by the boards (almost always an ACPE-accredited program) for a candidate to be eligible to take the state licensing examination. A listing of accredited professional programs offered by colleges and schools of pharmacy is published annually by ACPE and is available on the ACPE Web site (www.acpe-accredit.org).

Entering Practice and Updating Professional Knowledge and Skills

- Credentials earned: Licensure as registered pharmacist (R.Ph.); relicensure.
- Credential awarded by: State board of pharmacy
- Licensure process overseen by: State regulatory authorities

Before a graduate of a school or college of pharmacy can practice pharmacy in the United States, he or she must become licensed. The licensure process is regulated at the state level by the boards of pharmacy.

Candidates for licensure in all states but California must pass the North American Pharmacist Licensure Examination (NAPLEX), a computer-adaptive, competency-based examination that assesses the candidate's ability to apply knowledge gained in pharmacy school to real-life practice situations. California administers a unique examination process. Most states also require candidates to take a state-specific pharmacy law examination. Currently, 36 states use the Multistate Pharmacy Jurisprudence Examination (MPJE), a computer-adaptive assessment that tailors each examination to address the pharmacy law and regulations of the state in which the candidate is seeking licensure.

Both the NAPLEX and the MPJE are developed by the National Association of Boards of Pharmacy (NABP) for use by the boards of pharmacy as part of their assessment of competence to practice pharmacy. Development of these examinations is directly related to NABP's mission, which is to assist its member boards and jurisdictions in developing, implementing, and enforcing uniform standards for the purpose of protecting the public health. The NAPLEX and MPJE examinations are administered by appointment, daily, throughout the year at a system of test centers located in all 50 states.

In addition to the NAPLEX and MPJE, some states require a laboratory examination or an oral examination before licensure is conferred. All state boards also require that candidates complete an internship before being licensed. The internship may be completed during the candidate's academic training or after graduation, depending upon state requirements.

State licensure is an indication that the individual has attained the basic degree of competence necessary to ensure the public health and welfare will be reasonably well protected. Individuals who have received a license may use the abbreviation "R.Ph." (for "registered pharmacist") after their names.

Nearly all state boards of pharmacy also require that registered pharmacists complete a certain number of continuing-education units (CEUs) before they can renew their licenses. The CEUs must be earned through participation in a continuing-education (CE) program whose provider has been approved by the American Council on Pharmaceutical Education (ACPE). The symbol used by ACPE to designate that the CE provider is approved is ![AC PE logo].

Note that ACPE approves providers of CE, not individual CE programs. CEUs may be secured by attending educational seminars, teleconferences, and meetings; reading journal articles; or completing traditional home study courses or computer-based education programs. Receipt of a satisfactory score on an assessment that is created by and submitted to the CE provider is sometimes required as a documentation of completion of a CE program. ACPE publishes an annual directory of approved providers of continuing pharmaceutical education, which is available on the ACPE Web site (www.acpe-accredit.org).

Licensure and relicensure are mandatory for pharmacists who wish to continue to practice their profession.

In their regulatory role, state boards of pharmacy are ultimately responsible to the state legislature.

Developing and Enhancing Knowledge and Skills

Pharmacy practitioners who wish to broaden and deepen their knowledge and skills may participate in a variety of postgraduate education and training opportunities. They include the following:

Academic Postgraduate Education and Training

Pharmacists who wish to pursue a certain field of study in depth may enroll in postgraduate master's or doctor of philosophy (Ph.D.) programs. Common fields of study for master's candidates include business administration, clinical pharmacy, and public health. Common fields for Ph.D. studies include pharmacology, pharmaceutics, pharmacy practice, and social and administrative sciences.

Residencies

- Credential earned: Residency certificate
- Credential awarded by: Residency training program
- Program accreditation: The American Society of Health-System Pharmacists (ASHP) (independently or in collaboration with other pharmacy organizations)

ASHP is the chief accreditation body for pharmacy practice and specialty residency programs in pharmacy. A total of 505 programs nationwide now hold ASHP accreditation. ASHP also partners with other organizations, including the Academy of Managed Care Pharmacy, the American College of Clinical Pharmacy, the American Pharmaceutical Association, and the American Society of Consultant Pharmacists, in accrediting residency programs.

The majority of pharmacists who pursue residency training do so in the area of pharmacy practice. These residencies sometimes focus on a particular practice setting, such as ambulatory care. Pharmacists may also pursue specialty training in a certain topic (e.g., pharmacokinetics), in the care of a specific patient population (e.g., pediatrics), or in a specific disease area (e.g., oncology).

Residency programs last one to two years. The typical training site is a practice setting such as an academic health center, a community pharmacy, a managed care organization, a skilled nursing facility, or a home health care agency.

The Health Care Financing Administration (HCFA), an agency of the federal government, recognizes residency accreditation bodies within the health professions.

Fellowships[a]

- Credential earned: Fellowship certificate
- Credential awarded by: Fellowship training program
- Program accreditation: No official accreditation body

A fellowship is an individualized postgraduate program that prepares the participant to become an independent researcher. Fellowship programs, like residencies, usually last one to two years. The programs are developed by colleges of pharmacy, academic health centers, colleges and universities, and pharmaceutical manufacturers.

There is no official accreditation body for fellowship programs; however, the American Association of Colleges of Pharmacy and American College of Clinical Pharmacy have issued guidelines that are followed by many fellowship program directors.

Certificate Training Programs

- Credential earned: Certificate of Completion
- Credential awarded by: Educational institutions and companies, pharmacy organizations, and others
- Provider accreditation: American Council on Pharmaceutical Education

A certificate training program is a structured and systematic postgraduate continuing-education experience for pharmacists that is generally smaller in magnitude and shorter in duration than degree programs. Certificate programs are designed to instill, expand, or enhance practice competencies through the systematic acquisition of specified knowledge, skills, attitudes, and behaviors. The

focus of certificate programs is relatively narrow; for example, the American Pharmaceutical Association offers programs in such areas as asthma, diabetes, immunization delivery, and management of dyslipidemias.

Certificate training programs are offered by national and state pharmacy organizations and by schools and colleges of pharmacy and other educational groups. The programs are often held in conjunction with a major educational meeting of an organization. The American Council on Pharmaceutical Education (ACPE) approves providers of such programs. The symbol used by the ACPE to designate that a certificate training program is provided by an accredited provider is (P) ACPE.

Traineeships

Traineeships, in contrast to certificate training programs, are defined as intensive, individualized, structured postgraduate programs intended to provide the participant with the knowledge and skills needed to provide a high level of care to patients with various chronic diseases and conditions. Traineeships are generally of longer duration (about five days) and involve smaller groups of trainees than certificate training programs do. Some are offered on a competitive basis, with a corporate sponsor or other organization underwriting participants' costs. Pharmacy organizations currently offering traineeships include the American College of Apothecaries, the American Society of Consultant Pharmacists, and the American Society of Health-System Pharmacists Research and Education Foundation.

Certification

Introduction

Certification is a credential granted to pharmacists and other health professionals who have demonstrated a level of competence in a specific and relatively narrow area of practice

that exceeds the minimum requirements for licensure. Certification is granted on the basis of successful completion of rigorously developed eligibility criteria that include a written examination and, in some cases, an experiential component. The certification process is undertaken and overseen by a nongovernmental body.

The development of a certification program includes the following steps:

- *Role delineation.* The first step is to define the area in which certification is to be offered. This is done through a process called role delineation or "task analysis." An expert panel of individuals in the proposed subject area develops a survey instrument to assess how practitioners working in the area rate the importance, frequency, and criticality of specific activities in that practice. The instrument is then sent to a sample of pharmacists who are practicing in that field.
- *Development of content outline.* On the basis of responses to the survey, a content outline for the certification program is developed.
- *Preparation of examination.* The written examination component of the certification program is developed on the basis of the content outline.
- *Other activities.* Appropriate measures are taken to ensure that security and confidentiality of the testing process are maintained, that the examination and eligibility criteria are appropriate, and that the knowledge and skills of those who are certified do, in fact, reflect competence.

A professional testing company typically assists in the development of the role delineation and the examination to ensure that the examination meets professional standards of psychometric soundness and legal defensibility.

Certifying Agencies for Pharmacists Only

Three groups—the Board of Pharmaceutical Specialties, the Commission for Certification in Geriatric Pharmacy, and the National Institute for Standards in Pharmacist Credentialing—offer certification to pharmacists.

Board of Pharmaceutical Specialties (BPS). Established in 1976 by the American Pharmaceutical Association, BPS is the only agency that offers certification at the specialty level in pharmacy. It certifies pharmacists in five specialties: nuclear pharmacy, nutrition support pharmacy, oncology pharmacy, pharmacotherapy, and psychiatric pharmacy. As of January 2000, nearly 3000 pharmacists held BPS certification, distributed across the five specialties as follows:

1. Nuclear Pharmacy—444
2. Nutrition Support Pharmacy—451
3. Oncology Pharmacy—184
4. Pharmacotherapy—1546
5. Psychiatric Pharmacy—311

Pharmacists who wish to retain BPS certification must be recertified every seven years.

The recognition of each specialty is the result of a collaborative process between the Board and one or more pharmacy organizations, which develop a petition to support and justify recognition of the specialty. This petition must meet written criteria established by the BPS.

The BPS is directed by a nine-member board that includes six pharmacists, two health professionals who are not pharmacists, and one public/consumer member. A specialty council of six specialist members and three pharmacists not in the specialty direct the certification process for each specialty.

BPS examinations are administered with the assistance of an educational testing firm, resulting in a process that is psychometrically sound and legally defensible. Each of the five specialties has its own eligibility criteria, examination specifications, and recertification process. All five examinations are given on a single day once a year in approximately 25 sites in the United States and elsewhere.

In 1997, BPS introduced a method designed to recognize focused areas within pharmacy specialties. A designation of "Added Qualifications" denotes that an individual has demonstrated an enhanced level of training and experience in one segment of a BPS-recognized specialty. Added qualifications are conferred on the basis of a portfolio review to qualified individuals who already hold BPS certification. The first added qualification to receive BPS approval was infectious diseases, within the pharmacotherapy specialty.

Commission for Certification in Geriatric Pharmacy (CCGP). In 1997, the American Society of Consultant Pharmacists (ASCP) Board of Directors voted to create the CCGP to oversee a certification program in geriatric pharmacy practice. CCGP is a nonprofit corporation that is autonomous from ASCP. It has its own governing Board of Commissioners. The CCGP Board of Commissioners includes five pharmacist members, one physician member, one payer/employer member, one public/consumer member, and one liaison member from the ASCP Board of Directors.

Pharmacists who meet CCGP's requirements are entitled to use the designation Certified Geriatric Pharmacist, or CGP. As of January 2000, approximately 400 pharmacists have earned the CGP credential. Pharmacists who wish to retain their CGP credential must recertify every five years by successfully completing a written examination.

CCGP contracts with a professional testing firm to assist in conducting the role delineation or task analysis and in developing and administering the examination. The resulting process is psychometrically sound and legally defensible; it also meets nationally recognized standards. The CGP certification exams are administered twice a year at multiple locations in the United States, Canada, and Australia. CCGP publishes a candidate handbook that includes the content outline for the examination, eligibility criteria for taking the examination, and the policies and procedures of the certification program.

National Institute for Standards in Pharmacist Credentialing (NISPC). The NISPC was founded in 1998 by the American Pharmaceutical Association, the National Association of Boards of Pharmacy (NABP), the National Association of Chain Drug Stores, and the National Community Pharmacists Association. The purpose of NISPC is to "promote the value and encourage the adoption of National Association of Boards of Pharmacy disease-specific examinations as the consistent and objective means of documenting the ability of pharmacists to provide disease state management services."

NISPC offers certification in the management of diabetes, asthma, dyslipidemia, and anticoagulation therapy. At the time of its founding, the organization's immediate objective was to design a process that would document the competence of pharmacists providing care for patients with these disease states. The NISPC credential was first recognized in the state of Mississippi, where it was used to enable pharmacists to qualify for Medicaid reimbursement as part of a pilot project in that state. NABP developed the competency assessment examinations and oversees their administration. As of May 2000, 1089 pharmacists hold NISPC certification: 653 in diabetes, 227 in asthma, 110 in dyslipidemia, and 99 in anticoagulation therapy.

The NISPC tests are administered nationally as computerized examinations and are available throughout the year.

Multidisciplinary Certification Programs

Some certification programs are available to professionals from many health disciplines, including pharmacists. Areas in which such certification is available include diabetes education, anticoagulation therapy, pain management, and asthma education. Some of these programs are still in the early stages of development. Several of these providers are listed in Appendix B; however, the information is not intended to be exhaustive.

PHARMACY SUPPORTIVE PERSONNEL

A pharmacy technician is an individual who assists in pharmacy activities that do not require the professional judgment of a pharmacist. For example, pharmacy technicians may accept orders from patients, prepare labels, enter drug information into the pharmacy's computer system, and retrieve medications from inventory. As pharmacists assume an increasing number of clinical roles, pharmacy technicians are taking more and more responsibility for distributive functions in pharmacies in all settings.

The exact functions and responsibilities of pharmacy technicians are defined by state laws and regulations and are also determined by the willingness of pharmacists to delegate the nonjudgmental activities of their practice. Pharmacy technicians always work under the supervision of a licensed pharmacist.

The education and training, certification, and continuing education of pharmacy technicians are similar in some ways to those of pharmacists.

Education and Training

Most pharmacy technicians today have been trained on the job, either formally or informally. As the responsibilities of pharmacy technicians grow, however, more and more individuals are enrolling in formal training programs. These programs are generally affiliated with a community college, a four-year college, a hospital, or another health care organization. Graduates of these programs may be awarded an associate's degree or a certificate of completion.

ASHP is the accreditation body for pharmacy technician training programs. Sixty programs were accredited as of 1999.

Regulation

State boards of pharmacy oversee the registration of pharmacy technicians. Practices differ substantially from state to state.

Certification

The Pharmacy Technician Certification Board (PTCB) was established in 1995 as a national voluntary certification program for pharmacy technicians. Its founders were the American Pharmaceutical Association, the American Society of Health-System Pharmacists, the Illinois Council of Health-System Pharmacists, and the Michigan Pharmacists Association.

In collaboration with testing experts, the PTCB developed a national examination, the Pharmacy Technician Certification Examination (PTCE). The examination is designed to assess the candidate's knowledge and skill base for activities that are most commonly performed by a pharmacy technician, as determined by a national task analysis.

The Board administers the PTCE three times a year at more than 120 sites across the nation. A technician who passes the PTCE is designated as a Certified Pharmacy Technician (CPhT). More than 60,000 pharmacy technicians have earned PTCB certification.

Pharmacy technicians must renew their certification every two years. To qualify for recertification, they must participate in at least 20 hours of pharmacy-related continuing education that includes an hour of pharmacy law.

---

[a] Several pharmacy organizations, including the American College of Clinical Pharmacy, the American Society of Health-System Pharmacists, and the American Pharmaceutical Association, award the honorary title of "Fellow" to selected members as a means of publicly recognizing their contributions to the profession. A Fellow of ASHP, for example, may write "FASHP" for "Fellow of the American Society of Health-System Pharmacists" after his or her name. The two uses of the word "fellow"—one denoting an individual participating in a postgraduate training program and the other denoting receipt of an honorary title—should be clearly distinguished.

Appendix A—Glossary[a]

Accreditation: The process whereby an association or agency grants public recognition to an organization that meets certain established qualifications or standards, as determined through initial and periodic evaluations.

Certificate: A certificate is a document issued to a pharmacist upon successful completion of the predetermined level of performance of a certificate training program or of a pharmacy residency or fellowship. See also "statement of continuing-education credit."

Certificate Training Program: A structured, systematic postgraduate education and continuing-education experience for pharmacists that is generally smaller in magnitude and shorter in duration than a degree program. Certificate programs are designed to instill, expand, or enhance practice competencies through the systematic acquisition of specific knowledge, skills, attitudes, and performance behaviors.

Certification: The voluntary process by which a nongovernmental agency or association formally grants recognition to a pharmacist who has met certain predetermined qualifications specified by that organization. This recognition designates to the public that the holder has attained the requisite level of knowledge, skill, or experience in a well-defined, often specialized, area of the total discipline. Certification entails assessment, including testing, an evaluation of the candidate's education and experience, or both. Periodic recertification is usually required to retain the credential.

Certified: Adjective that is used to describe an individual who holds certification and that is incorporated into the name of the credential awarded that individual. For example, someone who has earned BPS certification in oncology is a "Board-Certified Oncology Pharmacist."

Clinical Privileges: Authorization to provide a specific range of patient care services. See "privileging."

Competence: The ability to perform one's duties accurately, make correct judgments, and interact appropriately with patients and with colleagues. Professional competence is characterized by good problem-solving and decision-making abilities, a strong knowledge base, and the ability to apply knowledge and experience to diverse patient-care situations.

Competency: A distinct skill, ability, or attitude that is essential to the practice of a profession. Individual competencies for pharmacists include, for example, mastery of aseptic technique and achievement of a thought process that enables one to identify therapeutic duplications. A pharmacist must master a variety of competencies in order to gain competence in his or her profession.

Continuing Education: Organized learning experiences and activities in which pharmacists engage after they have completed their entry-level academic education and training. These experiences are designed to promote the continuous development of the skills, attitudes, and knowledge needed to maintain proficiency, provide quality service or products, respond to patient needs, and keep abreast of change.

Credential: Documented evidence of professional qualifications. For pharmacists, academic degrees, state licensure, and Board certification are all examples of credentials.

Credentialing: (1) The process by which an organization or institution obtains, verifies, and assesses a pharmacist's qualifications to provide patient care services. (2) The process of granting a credential (a designation that indicates qualifications in a subject or an area).

Fellowship: A directed, highly individualized postgraduate program designed to prepare a pharmacist to become an independent researcher.

License: A credential issued by a state or federal body that indicates that the holder is in compliance with minimum mandatory governmental requirements necessary to practice in a particular profession or occupation.

Licensure: The process of granting a license.

Pharmacy Technician: An individual who, under the supervision of a licensed pharmacist, assists in pharmacy activities not requiring the professional judgment of the pharmacist.

Privileging: The process by which a health care organization, having reviewed an individual health care provider's credentials and performance and found them satisfactory, authorizes that individual to perform a specific scope of patient care services within that organization.

Registered: Adjective used to describe a pharmacist who has met state requirements for licensure and whose name has been entered on a state registry of practitioners who are licensed to practice in that jurisdiction.

Residency: An organized, directed, postgraduate training program in a defined area of pharmacy practice.

Scope of Practice: The boundaries within which a health professional may practice. For pharmacists, the scope of practice is generally established by the board or agency that regulates the profession in a given state or organization.

Statement of Continuing-Education Credit: A document issued to a pharmacist upon completion of a continuing-education program provided by an organization approved by the American Council on Pharmaceutical Education

Traineeship: A short, intensive, clinical and didactic postgraduate educational program intended to provide the pharmacist with knowledge and skills needed to provide a high level of care to patients with specific diseases or conditions.

---

*These definitions have been developed by a variety of organizations involved in credentialing and are generally accepted by those in the pharmacist credentialing arena.

Appendix B—Referenced Pharmacy Organizations and Certification Bodies

Pharmacy Organizations

Academy of Managed Care Pharmacy (AMCP)
100 North Pitt Street, Suite 400
Alexandria, VA 22314
(800) 827-2627
www.amcp.org

American Association of Colleges of Pharmacy (AACP)
1426 Prince Street
Alexandria, VA 22314-2841
(703) 836-8982
www.aacp.org

American College of Apothecaries (ACA)
P.O. Box 341266
Memphis, TN 38184
www.acaresourcecenter.org

American College of Clinical Pharmacy (ACCP)
3101 Broadway, Suite 380
Kansas City, MO 64111
(816) 531-2177
www.accp.com

American Council on Pharmaceutical Education (ACPE)
311 W. Superior Street, Suite 512
Chicago, IL 60610
(312) 664-3575
www.acpe-accredit.org

American Pharmaceutical Association (APhA)
2215 Constitution Avenue, NW
Washington, DC 20037-2985
(202) 628-4410
www.aphanet.org

American Society of Consultant Pharmacists (ASCP)
1321 Duke Street
Alexandria, VA 22314-3563
(703) 739-1300
www.ascp.com

American Society of Health-System Pharmacists (ASHP)
7272 Wisconsin Avenue
Bethesda, MD 20814
(301) 657-3000
www.ashp.org

National Association of Boards of Pharmacy (NABP)
700 Busse Highway
Park Ridge, IL 60068
(847) 698-6227
www.nabp.net

National Association of Chain Drug Stores (NACDS)
413 N. Lee Street, P.O. Box 1417-D49
Alexandria, VA 22313-1480
(703) 549-3001
www.nacds.org

National Community Pharmacists Association (NCPA)
205 Daingerfield Road
Alexandria, VA 22314
(703) 683-8200
www.ncpanet.org

Certification Bodies for Pharmacists or Pharmacy Technicians (May be multidisciplinary)

Anticoagulation Forum
88 East Newton Street, E-113
Boston, MA 02118-2395
(617) 638-7265
www.acforum.org

Board of Pharmaceutical Specialties (BPS)
2215 Constitution Avenue, NW
Washington, DC 20037-2985
(202) 429-7591
www.bpsweb.org

Council on Certification in Geriatric Pharmacy (CCGP)
1321 Duke Street
Alexandria, VA 22314-3563
(703) 535-3038
www.ccgp.org

National Asthma Educator Certification Board
American Lung Association
1740 Broadway
New York, NY 10019-4374
(212) 315-8865
www.lungusa.org

National Certification Board for Diabetes Educators (NCBDE)
330 East Algonquin Road, Suite 4
Arlington Heights, IL 60005
(847) 228-9795
www.nbcde.org

National Institute for Standards in Pharmacist Credentialing (NISPC)
P.O. Box 1910
Alexandria, VA 22313-1910
(703) 299-8790
www.nispcnet.org

Pharmacy Technician Certification Board (PTCB)
2215 Constitution Avenue, NW
Washington, DC 20037-2985
(202) 429-7576
www.ptcb.org

Practical Approaches to Collecting Outcomes in Pharmacy Practice

Steve Riddle, Marianne Weber

CHAPTER
23

Tracking quality measures and exploring outcomes in pharmacy practice improve patient care through the evaluation of current clinical practices. Appraising outcomes also provides data to support the value of clinical pharmacy programs and pharmacists. While the positive impact of clinical pharmacy services on cost and health-related outcomes has been well documented in the literature, it is often difficult for an individual institution or practice group to determine the value of this relationship. This is especially challenging in a collaborative practice model environment, where attributing a degree of benefit to a particular member of the health care team is difficult. Clinical pharmacists are an expensive investment, and it is critical that their value within both practice and the organization is demonstrated. In this chapter, we describe possible approaches for collecting data and demonstrating outcomes, which reflect the impact of clinical pharmacists' services.

Ways to define and classify outcomes in health care are numerous. Our department collects data from clinical pharmacist activities and interventions with patients and providers and translates it into reportable outcomes. We categorize the data in terms of quantitative and quality measures.

Quantitative Measures

Quantitative measures do not sufficiently reflect quality. However, while quantitative data may be perceived to have less value than its qualitative counterpart, the information is important for staff and administrators. For example, quantitative data are useful in assessing staff productivity and the cost effectiveness of medications.

257

Staff Productivity

In contrast to subjective reporting of activities, the measures that describe routine pharmacist functions provide useful objective data. These metrics help in determining the value of time spent on interventions or tasks. By evaluating the total time documented by staff versus the budgeted full-time equivalents (FTE), pharmacists can develop a crude productivity assessment. Quantitative information is, therefore, valuable to staff by providing a method of assessing activities and prioritizing job functions. It also enables pharmacy managers to communicate clinical activities to hospital administrators through regular and standardized reporting.

Cost-Effective Medication Use

Cost-related data, such as use of less expensive but clinically appropriate medications, are another important quantitative measure. While quantitative cost outcomes do not reflect quality of care, they carry significant weight in today's high-cost health care environment. Several cost measures that demonstrate the beneficial impact of the collaboration between pharmacists and providers include medication cost-per-patient, prescription, clinic, and disease state. Generic utilization rates are another common cost outcome. These rates can be tracked internally and are often benchmarked with similar organizations or compared to national averages. This comparative information is available on the Internet (e.g., Express Scripts Annual Drug Trend Report at www.express-scripts.com under news/industry reports) and from contracted third-party payers.

Engaging pharmacists to proactively influence physician prescribing behavior is a successful method of cost containment. Active involvement in promoting therapeutic substitution initiatives approved by Pharmacy and Therapeutics Committees, and the development and utilization of a preferred drug formulary also contribute to improved cost outcomes. At HMC, each primary care clinic has one or more clinical pharmacist specialists (CPS) who educate providers regarding the appropriate and safe use of cost-effective therapies, thus contributing to the success of these programs. In our experience, implementation of a preferred drug formulary saved an estimated $1 million in the first year with over $500,000 coming from five heavily targeted therapeutic groups (**Figure 23-1**). Cost-per-prescription is a measure that demonstrates the value of pharmacist involvement in promoting cost-effective medication utilization. **Figure 23-2** illustrates that our prescription costs are not only significantly lower than national averages, but have remained flat even after including inflation-related changes.

Quality Measures

Current outcomes assessments often classify quality measures using a progressive scale that includes care process measures, surrogate or interim clinical markers, and health outcomes measures. Many examples of these quality measures are available on the Internet or from quality improvement or oversight organizations such as the Centers for Medicare and Medicaid Services (CMS), the Joint Commission®, and the National Committee for Quality Assurance (NCQA) and their Health Plan Employer Data and Information Set (HEDIS). For information on CMS quality measures, which also includes links to non-CMS quality measure information, visit http://www.cms.hhs.gov/HospitalQualityInits/10_HospitalQualityMeasures.asp.

PDF Class	Volume Adjusted Cost Savings FY04	% use of PDF Agents		Average Cost per Rx	
		Pre-PDF	Post-PDF	Pre-PDF	Post-PDF
Nonsedating Antihistamines	$156,000	44%	74%	$34	$13
Long-acting Opioids	$203,000	30%	83%	$65	$35
Statins	$87,500	0%	33%	$50	$43
SSRIs	$61,000	34%	48%	$40	$33
Calcium Channel Blockers	$46,000	15%	18%	$44	$39
Totals	$553,500	25%	51%	$47	$33

Figure 23-1. UW Medicine Preferred Drug Formulary (PDF) Cost and Utilization Impact (selected examples)

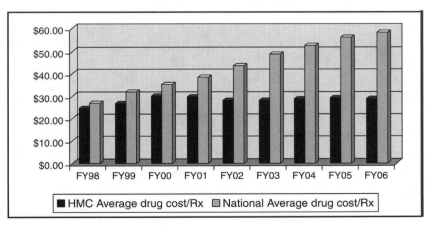

Figure 23-2. Harborview Medical Center Cost per Prescription Trends

Quality measures indicate direct or indirect improvements in care. Even in controlled clinical trials, determining the factors responsible for a given clinical outcome is challenging. In a real-world health care environment, this is even more difficult. Another challenge in a multidisciplinary, collaborative care model is determining which health outcomes are directly attributable to pharmacists. In our experience, most clinical quality measures are tracked in situations where the pharmacist is integrated into the care team. Examining specific measures focusing primarily on medication or medication-related outcomes is critical. Each chapter in this handbook includes goals of therapy or outcomes measures that are specific for the disease state co-managed by the clinical pharmacists. Whether or not a patient has met these goals is communicated to other members of the care team through documentation in the electronic medical record at every patient encounter.

Care Process Measures

Care process measures verify whether or not patients are being appropriately screened, monitored, and managed according to institutional policy and evidence-based guidelines. Examples include documentation of yearly screening for microalbuminuria and routine foot exams for patients with diabetes as well as annual lipid profiles for patients with coronary artery disease. These measures are considered lower level quality indicators because they do not assure a quality outcome, but they *do* indicate that key processes of care are being performed. For example, simply measuring LDL does not mean it is being properly evaluated or treated. Pharmacists can be key players assuring care process measures by recommending initiation of evidence-based medications (e.g., ACE inhibitors in systolic heart failure) or completion of tests for assessing drug safety and effectiveness (e.g., blood pressure checks at each office visit for patients with hypertension or hemoglobin A1C values every 3 months for patients with diabetes).

Surrogate Clinical Markers

Surrogate clinical markers are closely related to process measures, but of a higher quality. They describe whether or not a patient has met a predetermined goal of therapy that has been shown to impact health-related outcomes. From a pharmacy perspective, these markers are often drug-related outcome measures. Examples include the percent of INR values within the goal range for patients receiving warfarin or the number of patients with diabetes on hypoglycemic therapies achieving an HbA1C <7%.

Numerous opportunities exist for care improvements initiated by pharmacists related to surrogate clinical markers. We experienced success with a project designed to evaluate and improve adherence to CMS care process measures for heart failure. Baseline rates for use of evidence-based medications and ejection fraction measurements were collected on patients diagnosed with systolic heart failure, identified by the appropriate ICD-9 codes. Pharmacists targeted interventions with patients and providers to ensure compliance with recommended therapies. Data collection was repeated with benefits noted in the appropriate use of ACE inhibitors, beta-blockers, angiotensin receptor blockers, and improvements in left ventricular function (**Figure 23-3**).

Health Outcome Measures

The gold standard for determining value is health outcome measures, which include resource utilization (e.g., hospitalizations, emergency room visits) and morbidity and mortality. While they are common endpoints for controlled clinical trials, this level of information is difficult to obtain in ambulatory care settings due to the requirement for long-term follow-up and access to medical information. Therefore, these measures are often inferred based on how well the surrogate clinical and care process markers have been met using information published from large clinical trials. As an illustration, a CPS in 2001 participated in the Washington State Diabetes Collaborative. Seventy-four patients were referred to the pharmacist from one of four attending physicians for intensive diabetes care co-management, including medication adjustment, monitoring, and patient education. After 1 year, the patients who had been co-managed by the CPS had average HbA1C levels that were 1% lower than those receiving usual care (**Figure 23-4**). According to the National Institutes of Health Diabetes Control and Complications Trial (DCCT),[1] for every 1% decrease in HbA1C, the relative risk for microvascular complications decreases by 37%; diabetes-related deaths decrease by 21%; and myocardial infarction decreases by 14% (borderline significance). It would be impossible to demonstrate these important health outcomes for 74 patients over the course of 1 year; however by applying published data, a surrogate marker such as HbA1C becomes powerful information.

While health outcomes are difficult to capture, opportunities exist for pharmacists to generate this type of data in routine clinical practice. An anticoagulation management service, for example, may report rates of thromboembolism, episodes of clinically significant bleeding, and resource utilization (e.g., hospitalization).

Pharmacoeconomic Evaluations

Pharmacoeconomics is defined as the description and analysis of the costs and consequences of pharmaceutical products and/or services and their impact on individuals, health care systems, and society.[2] This definition includes both drug costs and the evaluation of services. Any economic evaluation model of clinical pharmacy services should consider and measure both costs and consequences. Schumock[3] describes three strategies for performing this assessment: 1) literature generalization, 2) economic modeling, and 3) local assessment. Literature generalization refers to application of published outcomes from sites similar to one's own. For example, when seeking to initiate pharmacy-based anticoagulation in a large, urban ambulatory care clinic, pharmacoeconomic data based on a service model for a similar setting would be valuable.

Criteria for Evaluation	Pre-Intervention	Post-Intervention	Goals
• Documented LVEF	89%	97%	>90%
• Beta-blocker therapy	65%*	79%*	>80%*
Patients with EF <40%			
• ACEI therapy	83%	100%	100%
• ACEI @ target dose	55%	73%	>90%
• ARB therapy (in patients with contraindications to ACEIs)	—	100%	100%

*Denominator includes patients with contraindications.

Figure 23-3. Impact of Pharmacist on Evidence-Based Care for Heart Failure

Measure	Initial Contact (Baseline)	1-Year Follow-Up
HbA1c (mean)	9.3%	8.2%
Self-management goal	27%	66%
Foot exam	11.1%	69%
BP 130/85 or less (most recent BP documented)	51%	66%

*Population: 74 Adult Medicine Clinic patients. 3+ encounters; January 2000–2001

Figure 23-4. Measuring Success of Case Management in a Longitudinally Defined Population: The Impact of a Coordinated Health Care Team*

Pharmacoeconomic evaluations using economic modeling are complex and time consuming and require a certain level of expertise and familiarity in order to be properly applied. The most commonly used pharmacoeconomic models include cost-minimization, cost-of-illness, cost-effectiveness, cost-benefit, and cost-utility analysis. Several schools of pharmacy have programs devoted to pharmacy outcomes, furthering the knowledge of these principles and models.

Intervention Tracking Systems

Numerous methods are available to help pharmacists capture, track, and report clinical interventions. Options range from simple paper-based systems to elaborate computer models with associated databases. System selection is dependent on available resources and the type of information desired.

Paper-Based Systems

Paper-based systems are simple to implement and user-friendly. A form or tracking card is devised that targets desired activities with a method (usually a hash mark) for indicating pharmacist action and a standard approach for noting the time involved. Our organization experimented with several versions of forms, shown in **Figures 23-5, 23-6,** and **23-7.**

The forms are completed by each pharmacy or clinical service and data are submitted to pharmacy administration. Time intervals for reporting vary depending on departmental preferences and may be regular or intermittent. Interventions and outcomes that are key indicators of pharmacists' routine activities may require more regular reporting. However, if activity levels are relatively constant and baseline values have been established, intermittent reporting may be acceptable and reduce the documentation burden for staff. In addition, intermittent reporting may be appropriate for specific projects or focused data collection, such as quarterly medication utilization reviews.

Another consideration is how the tracking card is used. We experimented with using a new card for each patient intervention and with one card to capture multiple interventions for many patients. The multiple intervention, multiple patient approach ultimately proved to be more practical because many interventions were quick, informal consults and completing a separate card for each was time consuming.

Computer-Based Systems

Quantifi® from PharmacyOneSource® (originally called HealthProLink™) is an Internet-based intervention tracking system. Originally designed to document inpatient pharmacy clinical interventions, our ambulatory clinical pharmacists trialed the system in 2005. We collaborated with a company representative to adjust the data entry form to collect information pertinent to ambulatory care activities. The project leaders spent a significant amount of time determining what specific data points would be included. A 3-month trial was completed with all clinical pharmacist specialists, following an initial small group pilot.

During the trial, each clinical pharmacist recorded information for all interventions performed (e.g., type of appointment, intervention type, time spent) at computers located in his or her practice areas. While PDA/handheld data collection was possible, we did not utilize this option due to the prohibitive costs of purchasing PDAs for our pharmacists. Because the pharmacists are required to chart formal patient encounters in the patient's medical record and complete billing forms, Internet-based tracking added yet another level of documentation.

Seven broad intervention types were followed in order to classify 52 disease state-related interventions. This technology allowed us to capture the average number of interventions per month and the total time required to complete and document these interventions. The level of detail allowed us to discern the exact number of drug order clarification interventions provided by pharmacists in

Pharmacist Activity Documentation

| Pharmacist: Date: |
| Clinic: |

Activity Type (circle all that apply):

1. Drug Info   6. Add Drug
2. Therapeutic choice   7. DC Drug
3. Dose recommendation   8. Add/DC lab test
4. PDF switch   9. Adverse drug event
5. Therapeutic duplication   10. Drug allergy
*Other:_____

Activity initiated by:
☐ RPh   ☐ MD   ☐ Midlevel   ☐ RN   ☐ Other

Compliance with recommendation:
☐ Followed
☐ Not followed, MD justification acceptable to pharmacist
☐ Not followed, Pharmacist disagrees
☐ Not applicable

Outcome (check all that apply):
☐ Avoid adverse drug event
☐ Reduce drug cost   ☐ Increase drug cost
☐ Reduce care cost   ☐ Increase care cost
☐ Improve effectiveness   ☐ Education
☐ Other:_____

Time Involved:
☐ < 5 min   ☐ 6–10 min   ☐ 11–20 min   ☐ > 20 min

Comments on back:

Figure 23-5. Single Intervention Tracking Form

Month/Year:_____

DISTRIBUTION PHARMACY STATS

Activity	Week 1	Week 2	Week 3	Week 4	Week 5	Total
Refill authorization (# of Patients)						
Mediset fill/refills (# of Medisets)						

CLINICAL PHARMACIST STATS

Activity	Week 1	Week 2	Week 3	Week 4	Week 5	Total
Refill authorization (# of Patients)						
Pain-related Refill Auth (# of Patients)						
Anticoagulation (# visits)						
New Patient						
Follow-up						
Phone						

Figure 23-6. Data Reporting Form (Monthly)

Patient encounters	Mon	Tues	Wed	Thurs	Fri	Total
Number of patients seen as "tag-on" visit						
Number of patients seen as "walk-in" visit						
Number of appointments scheduled						
Number of appointments kept						
Number of telephone follow-ups						
Home Visits						
Reasons for Referral						
Anticoagulation						
Asthma/COPD						
CHF/MI/Angina						
Diabetes						
HAART						
Hypertension						
Lipid management						
OTC triage						
Pain management						
Smoking Cessation						
Travel Medicine						
Multiple diseases (more than one illness)						
All other disease state referrals						
Quality Assurance/Outcomes Review	Mon	Tues	Wed	Thurs	Fri	Total
Type of Visit						
Level 1 Pharmacist visit						
Patient education in groups/classes						
Consultation Outcome						
Recommendation given						
Recommendation NOT accepted						
Other services						
Refill authorization						
Mediset fill/refills						
Limited staff education (easy questions)						
Literature search/staff education (in-services and more than the easy question)						

Figure 23-7. Activity Documentation Form (Weekly)

a specific clinic during a particular time period. Of note, we used the system to primarily track quantitative data, but the system was also able to track quality measures. As a result of this project, we were able to provide more detailed data reporting about pharmacist interventions to our staff and hospital administrators. We were also able to identify areas of inconsistency between clinic sites and streamline areas of practice. Examples of the types of interventions tracked and some of the data reports that were generated by the project are provided in **Tables 23-1 and 23-2.**

Table 23-1. Report by Intervention Type (Abbreviated)

HMC Ambulatory RX Jan 2005 Interventions

Interventions		4WC	AMC	Children's	FMC	IMC	Madison (ID)	Ortho	Pio Square (Indigent Care)	Women's	Totals
Adverse Effect Eval											
	#	4	4	3	5	2	1	9	2	6	36
	Time (min)	10	45	25	20	0	60	45	25	85	315
AntiCoag											
	#	60	186	6	32	15		72	25	14	410
	Time (min)	1005	2002	85	410	330		1850	300	205	6187
Asthma											
	#		10	26	6	1			1	5	49
	Time (min)		100	280	55	30			10	135	610
CAD-MI											
	#	15	10		10	7			8		50
	Time (min)	120	95		50	45			55		365
CHF											
	#	10	22		4	3			7		46
	Time (min)	120	235		50	35			40		480
Coordination of Care											0
	#	89	19		25	10	4	23	2	9	181
	Time (min)	436	120		115	95	130	215	480	35	1626
COPD											
	#	1	10		2	3			24		40
	Time (min)	5	65		30	25			210		335
Depression											
	#		8		4	1	10		1	3	27
	Time (min)		55		25	25	75		10	45	235
Diabetes											
	#	1	58	1	58	26			4	14	162
	Time (min)	30	1195	25	1020	630			80	355	3335
Drug Info											
	#	18	53	26	14	11	14	6	22	35	199
	Time (min)	141	289	159	120	55	85	30	335	243	1457
Drug Tx Reco											
	#	9	35	11	29	22	6	8	13	10	143
	Time (min)	65	173	80	75	125	135	45	95	55	848
DVT Program											
	#				1	5					6
	Time (min)				20	180					200
Education Pat Counsel											
	#	7	22	14	23	9	14	11	20	4	124
	Time (min)	80	125	140	240	90	110	80	40	100	1005
Hypertension											
	#	13	41	2	23	7			20	3	109
	Time (min)	75	585	20	215	0			135	25	1055
ID (infect dx)											
	#		1	2	15	1	35	11		4	69
	Time (min)		10	15	110	0	350	205		23	713
Lipid Management											
	#	20	13		5	19			11	6	74
	Time (min)	135	90		30	130			80	35	500
Med Adherence/Edu											
	#	14	41	20	7	10	16		24	1	133
	Time (min)	95	800	175	120	110	175		250	0	1725
Pain Management											
	#	9	10		25			305	1	11	361
	Time (min)	80	75		550			5590	15	107	6417
Smoking Cessation											
	#	5	4		7	2			31	5	54
	Time (min)	110	100		110	5			800	60	1185
Travel Medicine											
	#		2	6		2				3	13
	Time (min)		40	235		50				60	385
Totals											
	#	288	591	121	333	164	135	456	236	140	2464
	Time (min)	2507	6199	1239	3365	1960	1120	8060	2960	1568	28978

Table 23-2. Internet-Based Tracking Report by Intervention Type per Clinic per Pharmacist

Clinic	Consult #	Consult Time (min)	Sched Appt #	Sched Appt Time (min)	Tag On #	Tag On Time (min)	Telephone #	Telephone Time (min)	Walk In #	Walk In Time (min)	Refill Auth #	Refill Auth Time (min)	Other #	Other Time (min)	Totals #	Totals Time (min)
4WC	28	310	47	803	4	100	35	284	18	240	118	852	18	259	268	2848
CPS1	18	185	23	333	4	100	30	244	17	225	75	463	10	175		
CPS2	10	125	24	470			5	40	1	15	43	389	8	84		
AMC	143	842	223	3740	10	140	87	594	93	855	201	1032	6	110	763	7313
CPS3	113	685	89	1190	5	70	35	212	55	400	141	720	1	45		
CPS4	29	147	83	1020	2	25	44	332	15	105	59	307	4	55		
CPS5	1	10	51	1530	3	45	8	50	23	350	1	5	1	10		
Children's	40	383	18	430	22	295	9	110	4	50	39	332	21	147	153	1747
CPS6	26	200	1	45	10	120	6	85	3	30	23	180	8	65		
CPS7	14	183	5	150	12	175	3	25	1	20	14	137	5	37		
CPS8			12	235							2	15	8	45		
Endocrine	9	165	10	300	16	145	9	60							44	670
FMC	46	470	28	720	31	555	141	1426	15	275	26	148	11	1080	298	4674
CPS9	45	465	14	340	31	555	132	1351	13	255	4	33	4	630		
CPS10	1	5	14	380			9	75	2	20	22	115	7	450		
Hepatology	16	235	8	190	3	45					25	125	14	70	66	665
CPS11			8	190	3	45					25	125	14	70		
IMC	23	535	53	1415	1	40							4	155	81	2145
CPS12			8	210												
CPS13	3	25	45	1205	1	40							4	155		
Madison	22	520	18	650	12	180			3	45	16	325			71	1720
CPS14	10	125	12	420	10	150			1	15	2	15				
CPS15	12	395	6	230	2	30			2	30	14	310				
Ortho	37	815			9	240	327	6405	29	550					402	8010
CPS16	36	785			4	70	113	3075	17	335						
CPS17	1	30			5	170	214	3330	12	215						
Pio Square	29	395	39	775	1	5							2	480	71	1655
CPS18	7	85	11	135	1	5							2	480		
CPS19	14	255	16	295												
CPS20	8	55	12	345												
Women's	65	417	22	600	13	210	40	562	10	145	178	1202	29	302	357	3438
CPS21	41	275	15	375	7	105	24	420	5	105	125	875	10	90		
CPS22	24	142	7	225	6	105	16	142	5	40	53	327	19	212		
Totals	449	4922	456	9323	106	1810	639	9381	172	2160	603	4016	105	2603	2574	34885

The greatest challenge found in implementing this Internet-based technology was the amount of time required for staff to document interventions. Despite an efficient data entry design process, staff spent an additional 30–60 minutes per day completing documentation. Resolutions included having staff document only on key, targeted interventions during limited time periods or to only report on standard intervention activities for set periods on a yearly basis (e.g., 1 month of data collection every 6 months). Another challenge was that the system was designed for inpatient pharmacy intervention tracking, not ambulatory pharmacy. Because these processes of care are distinct, the modifications of the system further increased the complexity of implementation and training.

Our organization also uses an anticoagulation database designed to track patient information and care, create notes, and generate outcomes data. Created in Microsoft® Access by an internal programmer in collaboration with a clinical pharmacist, it is a well designed, stand-alone database that would be easily replicated by any organization with the necessary resources. The database requires clinical pharmacist input of both demographic and clinical information. The outcomes information generated is both quantitative (e.g., number of visits, visits per day, number of new referrals) and qualitative. The quality reporting includes the following health outcomes measures: effectiveness (number and type of thromboembolic events), safety (number of bleeds and severity), and resource utilization (emergency room visits, hospitalization). The database also reports surrogate clinical markers such as percentage of INR values within the targeted range.

Comparison of Tracking Systems

The low cost and ease of implementation make a paper-based approach practical. It is an excellent way to test early ideas for intervention tracking. There is no need for an expensive computer system to support this process. However, while using a paper-based system can be simple and efficient on the front-end for clinical staff, it does have limitations. Tallying information or creating a spreadsheet of data can be cumbersome, and interpreting illegible handwriting can be difficult.

Pharmacy managers and staff may appreciate the ease of report generation and customization that a computer-based system can provide. Some computer databases may be linked to other electronic information systems, allowing for auto-population of data fields, such as patient demographic or lab information. Stand-alone databases are useful, especially if the clinical focus is narrow, and may be easier to implement as they require less integration with other systems. But these databases will probably still require the manual entry of data, which is time consuming.

Electronic systems also provide expanded functionality beyond outcomes tracking. For example, our anticoagulation database allows for generation of

Table 23-3. Internet-Based Tracking Implementation Data Comparison

Activity	Paper	Internet-based		
		Nov-08	Dec-08	Jan-09
Total Pharmacist Consults/Interventions	1120	3192*	2750*	3157
Total Pharmacist Time in Interventions (hrs)	280	551	535	587
# of Refill Authorizations	1240	713	619	768
Disease State Management				
Anticoag	448	295	397	410
Asthma/COPD	54	54	48	55
CHF/MI/CAD	5	5	9	6
Diabetes	157	167	143	175
Dx State Referrals	71	?	?	?
DVT Program	1	5	0	6
HAART Program	44	32	32	39
Hepatitis	12	33	34	50
Hypertension	81	102	77	76
Infectious Disease/Home Antibiotics	8	14	23	34
Iron stores tracking/Anemia	2	39	0	5
Lipids/Dyslipidemia	13	30	18	12
Mental Health	No Data	34	0	10
OTC Triage	13	15	8	11
Pain Management	371	218	225	361
Smoking Cessation	38	41	29	49
Travel Med	27	12	22	13
Clinical Activities				
Adverse Drug Reporting/management	No Data	41	36	33
Coordination of Care	No Data	320	207	216
Dose Adjustments/Therapeutic Reco	No Data	392	256	235
Drug Information	No Data	94	168	166
Drug Interaction	No Data	16	21	16
Expanded Access Program (HIV)	No Data	0	0	0
Faculty Activity/Inservices	No Data	4	0	4
Med Education/Adherence	No Data	80	112	69
Patient Assistance Programs	No Data	2	4	1
PDF Implementation	No Data	3	5	5
Prior Authorization	No Data	30	43	51

*Includes all primary and secondary interventions

customized chart/SOAP notes that are imported electronically into the medical record. Databases also allow for the creation of customized patient education or disease management information, such as an asthma action plan. Other systems may provide clerical functions such as appointment scheduling or the generation of printed prescriptions.

Table 23-3 outlines the differences between the levels of data detail captured with our initial paper-based method as compared to the Internet-based data collection system.

Summary

Quality is currently a primary focus in health care. Medication-related safety concerns, increasing drug costs, and the appropriate use of resources have moved pharmacy to the forefront of health care quality discussions. Efforts to improve care must result in measurable outcomes that reflect value. As pharmacists assume greater roles in the provision of clinical services, it is imperative that we demonstrate our importance in assuring quality outcomes. In a collaborative care environment, the pharmacist is *the* medication therapy expert. However, demonstrating quality outcomes in collaborative practices can prove challenging when attempting to attribute outcomes to specific team members.

In evaluating our clinical pharmacy services, we chose to capture quantitative and qualitative data using both a paper-based system and a computer-based approach. Regardless of method, the key considerations in evaluating value added by clinical pharmacists include:

- A focus on areas where evidence-based medication-related care opportunities exist.
- Establishment of quality targets.
- Determination of metrics: care process measures, surrogate clinical markers, or health outcomes measures.
- Collection of baseline data to assure pre- and post-intervention outcomes data.

Once data collection is completed and the analysis begins, the doors will open to the evaluation of clinical pharmacy services and the value of clinical pharmacy through improved patient care outcomes.

References

1. The Diabetes Control and Complications Trial Research Group. The effect of intensive treatment of diabetes on the development and progress of long-term complications in insulin-dependent diabetes mellitus. *N Engl J Med*. 1993; 329:977–86.

2. Bootman JL, Townsend RJ, McGhan WF. Introduction to Pharmacoeconomics. In: Bootman JL, Townsend RJ, McGhan WF, eds. *Principles of pharmacoeconomics*. 3rd ed. Cincinnati, OH: Harvey Whitney Books; 2005:1–19.

3. Schumock GT. Methods to assess the economic outcomes of clinical pharmacy services. *Pharmacotherapy*. 2000; 20(10 Pt 2):243S–52S.

Index

Cardiovascular disease, 21, 35

Care process measures, 260

Carvedilol, 76, 80

CD/4 cell count, 147–48, 153, 155

CDTM. *See* Collaborative drug therapy management

Celecoxib, 193

Centers for Disease Control and Prevention, 97

Centers for Medicare and Medicaid Services, 259, 260

CHARM-Added trial, 76

Chloroquine phosphate, 214

Chlorthalidone, 80

Cholesterol-binding resins, 16

Cholesterol goals, 22–23

Chondroitin, 194

Chronic non-malignant pain
  clinical pharmacy goals, 179
  indications, 177
  management, 178–79
  outcomes, 179–80
  patient information resources, 180
  therapeutic goals, 179

Chronic pain
  contract, 181
  informed consent, 182

Ciprofloxacin, 138, 142, 216

Citalopram, 153, 202

Clarithromycin, 170, 173, 174

Clegg, Cynthia A., v, 243–55

Climara, 132

Clomipramine, 202

Clonidine, 41

Clopidogrel, 16, 18

Codeine, 194

Cognitive behavioral therapy, 100

Cognitive services, vii

Cold turkey cessation, 100

Collaborative drug therapy management (CDTM), vii, 11
  at-risk patient identification, 6

definitions, 1–2
improvements, 7
legislative history, 2
marketing services, 6
needs assessment, 6
obstacles to, 2, 4–5
outcomes, 7
process for starting, 5–6
program development, 6
providing service, 6–7
resource allocation, 6
state status, 3–4, 5

Computer-based tracking systems, 263, 265–68

Condom use, 118

Congestive heart care plan, 87–88

Conventional insulin therapy, 48

Coronary artery disease (CAD), 51, 75
  case study, 18–19
  clinical pharmacy goals, 17–18
  indications, 15
  outcomes, 18
  patient information resources, 18
  pharmacotherapy to improve symptoms, 16
  pharmacotherapy to reduce mortality, 15–16
  risk factors, 22
  risk management, 17
  therapeutic goals, 17

Coronary heart disease. *See* Coronary artery disease

Cost containment, 258, 259

Council on Credentialing in Pharmacy, 243

Cox-II selective inhibitors, 78, 193

Crabb, Karen, 127–35

Creatinine clearance, 62

Credentialing in pharmacy, 248–55

Cromolyn, 92

Cromolyn sodium, 90

Cytochrome P450, 68

Cytotoxic drugs, 129

D

Dalteparin, 61, 62

Dapsone, 147

Darunavir, 147, 151

DeCaro, Vicki, 191–98

Deep vein thrombosis, 59

Depression
  clinical pharmacy goals, 205
  indications, 199–201
  management, 201–5
  outcomes, 205
  patient information resources, 205–6
  therapeutic goals, 205

Desipramine, 202

Diabetes mellitus, 69
  case study, 55–57
  clinical pharmacy goals, 53–54
  comorbid conditions management, 51–52
  indications, 45–46
  management, 46–51
  outcomes, 54
  patient information resources, 55
  self-management education, 50–51
  therapeutic goals, 53

Didanosine EC, 151

Digoxin, 77, 81–82

Diphtheria vaccination, 52, 209, 222

Disopyramide, 78

Diuretics, 76, 80–81

Docosahexaenoic acid (DHA), 28

Docusate, 185, 221

Doxycycline, 214, 223

Drug–disease interactions, 104

Drug–drug interactions, 68, 104, 148

Drug resistance, 150